JESUS HEALS

RECEIVE YOUR HEALING TODAY!

JOHN MAXWELL

Special thanks

All glory and honour to God! With special thanks to my beautiful wife, Yeng, my father and mother, John and Eileen Maxwell, the Chuah family, Charles Harbottle, Austin McDermott and David Goodship for all their love, help, support and prayers.

JESUS HEALS

ISBN: 9798370837241

Published 2023

Edited by Yeng Maxwell

Text copyright of John Maxwell 2023
All rights reserved. No part of this book may be reproduced, stored in a retrieval system or transmitted in any form or by means electronic, mechanical, photocopying or otherwise without the prior written consent of the writer.

Scripture quotations are based on the World English Bible (WEB) which is in the public domain. The WEB is a 1997 version of the American Standard Version of 1901.

CONTENTS

1	Jesus turned water into wine	7
2	Jesus healed an official's son	11
3	A miraculous catch of fish	13
4	Demoniac healed on a Sabbath	19
5	Jesus healed Peter's mother-in-law	23
6	Jesus healed all in Capernaum	27
7	Jesus healed a leper in Galilee	31
8	Jesus healed a paralytic	39
9	Jesus healed a man's hand	49
10	Centurion's servant healed	55
11	Jesus raised a widow's son	61
12	Jesus healed a blind mute	65
13	Jesus calmed a storm	69
14	Jesus healed two demoniacs	73
15	Jesus healed a bleeding woman	79
16	Jesus raised Jairus' daughter	87
17	Jesus healed two blind men	93
18	Jesus healed a mute demoniac	97
19	Paralytic healed in Jerusalem	101
20	Jesus fed the Five Thousand	105
21	Jesus walked on water	113
22	Demonised daughter healed in Tyre	123
23	Jesus healed a deaf mute	127
24	Jesus fed the Four Thousand	129
25	Blind man healed in Bethsaida	135
26	Blind man healed in Jerusalem	139
27	Jesus raised Lazarus	147
28	Jesus healed a demonised son	155
29	Miracle coin in a fish's mouth	161
30	Jesus healed ten lepers	163
31	Jesus healed a crippled woman	167
32	Jesus healed a man with dropsy	171
33	Jesus healed two blind men	175
34	Jesus cursed a fig tree	181
35	Jesus healed a man's ear	185
36	A miraculous catch of fish	187
	Jesus healed the crowds and Summary	193

Introduction

During his time on Earth Jesus, the Son of God preached the Good News of the kingdom of God, healed the sick and cast out demons. Jesus did so many miracles, John 21:25 says the world would not have enough room for all the books that would be written. Yet only thirty-six of Jesus' miracles are recorded in the Gospels. This shows the Gospel writers, inspired by the Holy Spirit recorded that number for a specific purpose. An examination of the thirty-six miracles will reveal what that purpose was and what it reveals about Jesus, his miracles and his healings and how they apply to us today.

'*Jesus Heals*' examines all the miracles he performed in thirty-six separate chapters. Each miracle reveals different aspects of the kingdom of God and the variety of ways in which Jesus performed his healings, signs and wonders. It shows the levels of faith and the different ways with which people came to Jesus for healing and will inspire us to approach him in faith for our healing today. Faith comes by hearing and hearing by the word of God. As we read the word of God and as we hear it and take it into our hearts, our souls and our bodies, it is spirit and it is life to us and it heals us.

For pastors, each chapter in the book can be used as a sermon. Some miracles and healings can be put together for a talk or series of talks. The book ends with a summary of the miracles. After looking at Jesus' miracles you may form your own conclusions. I pray that as you read this book, you will be healed even before you finish the book. If not, then keep on reading until you are healed.

May God bless you and heal you for his glory!

Miracle 1

Jesus turned water into wine

'On the third day a wedding took place at Cana in Galilee. Jesus' mother was there and Jesus and his disciples had also been invited to the wedding. When the wine was gone, Jesus' mother said to him, "They have no more wine."

"Dear woman, why do you involve me?" Jesus replied. "My time has not yet come."

His mother said to the servants, "Do whatever he tells you."

Nearby stood six stone water jars, the kind used by the Jews for ceremonial washing, each holding from twenty to thirty gallons. So, Jesus said to the servants, "Fill the jars with water"; so they filled them to the brim. Then he told them, "Now draw some out and take it to the master of the banquet."

They did so and the master of the banquet tasted the water that had been turned into wine. He did not realise where it had come from, but the servants who had drawn the water knew. Then he called the bridegroom aside and said, "Everyone brings out the choice wine first then the cheaper wine after the guests have had too much to drink; but you have saved the best till now."

This, the first of his miraculous signs, Jesus performed at Cana in Galilee. He thus revealed his glory; and his disciples put their faith in him.' – **John 2:1-11**

1. Jesus turned water into wine

Jesus performed his first miracle at a wedding he attended in Cana in Galilee. Mary, his mother learned the hosts had run out of wine. She brought this to Jesus' attention, because she believed he could solve the situation. Her idea of resolution could have been, Jesus would go to the nearest wine merchant and get enough wine to last until the end of the wedding celebration. His response was unusual. He asked Mary why she was involving him in this matter then he told her that his time had not yet come. Let's examine why Jesus responded to his mother Mary in this most unusual way.

Christian tradition suggests Joseph, Jesus' earthly father had died before he was baptised and his ministry began. As the oldest son, he would have taken over as the head of the household. Mary may have turned to him for help out of instinct, as it had been her habit since Joseph had passed away. Jesus was not rebuffing Mary's concerned approach. He was showing his mother this was the time when their relationship had to change. Jesus had to focus on the ministry that his heavenly Father had given him to do on planet Earth.

Listen to Jesus and obey him

Mary's answer is her last words recorded in the Gospels: *"Do whatever he tells you!"* (John 2:5). Her words to the servants at the wedding in Cana are the same words God speaks to us today. If Jesus tells us to do something, we must obey and do what he says. Mary's last words about Jesus are: *"Do whatever he tells you!"* His Father's last words about Jesus at the Transfiguration are, *"This is my Son, whom I love. Listen to him!"* (Mark 9:7). How wonderful! His mother and Father both said Jesus must be listened to. This was said at the beginning and the end of his ministry, so we must listen to Jesus from beginning to end, that is, for all our lives. Jesus' words are Spirit and they are life. We must listen to his words continually. When we listen and do what Jesus says then the water of life in our lives will turn into the fullness of the wine of the kingdom of God.

This miracle is a parable

The miracle of turning water into wine is a parable that contrasts grace and the Law. John 2:6 says six stone water jars, used for ceremonial washing stood nearby. The jars represent the Law, that is the Ten Commandments, written on tablets of stone. The jars were cold and empty like the Law. The Law is good, righteous and holy, but it cannot impart goodness, righteousness and holiness. Beside the jars stood grace in the person of Jesus. He filled the jars with warm, fruitful, colourful, intoxicating wine. This miracle contrasts the Old and New Covenant. Wine is tastier and more colourful than water. When we drink water it quenches our thirst, but we are unchanged. When we drink the wine of Jesus we come alive. We are born again. His wine brings a new thing into our lives, the New Birth. There is no condemnation in this life, as God accepts us in Christ Jesus.

The Law has been replaced. We are given one grace in place of another grace (John 1:16). It is like we are the seashore and grace is the waves relentlessly rolling onto shore, one after another. The Law is good, but something better replaced it. The Law came on tablets of stone. Grace came in the person of Jesus. This miracle represents the transition from Law to grace. The time of the law of condemnation and death was over and the time of grace, of no condemnation and of life had come. Jesus came to inaugurate a new way of living and believing.

The time of the Mosaic Law was over. The new era of the Spirit and of grace had come. The Law was good. It was grace from God. But Jesus introduced a new era, with a higher level of grace. It is the grace of the cross – of God's Son dying on the cross for our sins. It is the grace of the higher life – life in the Spirit and God's kingdom being established on Earth. It is the sweet wine of the New Birth. It is not life under the controlling Law. If you break the Law you die. Grace came to us in the person of Jesus. In him we are born again and will never die. It is not power outside us. It is power inside us. It is just like wine. It warms us inside and it stimulates us and warms us to the things of God.

Jesus' story begins with a wedding

It takes wine at a wedding to illustrate this. The Law came through Moses. Grace and truth came through Jesus. Grace is a person. Moses turned water into blood. Jesus turned water into wine. The manifestation of the Law is death. The manifestation of grace in the kingdom of God is life – eternal life. It is like a wedding, full of celebration and joy. It is the kingdom of New Wine. It gets better with age and it is a party that never ends. Life does not deteriorate in his kingdom but keeps on growing. It is life as a Christian. The Gospel of Jesus begins with a wedding and it ends with a wedding when Jesus marries forever, his bride – the Church and we will be filled with joy forever. In Genesis 24, Abraham sent out his faithful servant to find a bride for his son, Isaac. Today, God sends out his faithful servant, the Holy Spirit to seek a bride for Christ – the members of his Church. We will have eternal life in the presence of God the Father, where joy will overflow and never end.

Jesus is Lord of time and matter

Jesus' first miracle shows God is intimately interested in the details of our lives. He saved a wedding from disaster. It takes over seven years to produce wine – from the planting of the vines to bottling the wine. The best wines take longer to make, but Jesus produced the best wine in a moment. It shows he is Lord of time and Lord of substance and matter. This is life with Jesus. We do not have to wait. We can have the best of all he has now – be it love, provision, health, favour, healing and fullness of life in him. And it was servants at a wedding, not kings or priests who were first to see his miraculous powers as they filled the jars with water and served it as wine. Jesus chose the lowest class in society to be the first to see his divinity. This is Jesus. This is the Living God in human form. God announced His Son's birth first to shepherds (Luke 2:8-20). Today, he comes to us saying, we do not have to be successful or famous or perfect to receive his salvation or healing. He receives us as we are, no matter where we are coming from.

Miracle 2

Jesus healed an official's son

'Once more he visited Cana in Galilee where he had turned the water into wine. And there was a certain royal official whose son lay sick at Capernaum. When this man heard that Jesus had arrived in Galilee from Judea, he went to him and begged him to come and heal his son, who was close to death.

"Unless you people see miraculous signs and wonders," Jesus told him, "you will never believe."

The official said, "Sir, come down before my child dies."

Jesus replied, "You may go. Your son will live."

He took Jesus at his word and departed. While he was on the way, his servants met him with the news that his boy was living. When he inquired as to the time his son got better, they said to him, "The fever left him yesterday, at the seventh hour."

Then the father realised *it was the exact time at which Jesus had said to him, "Your son will live*." So he and his whole household believed.

This was the second miraculous sign that Jesus performed having come from Judea to Galilee.' – **John 4:46-54**

2. Jesus healed an official's son

The official believed Jesus had the power to heal his son, but only if he came to him. When he asked Jesus to heal his son, Jesus said, *"Unless you people see miraculous signs and wonders, you will never believe."* Like his first miracle, his response to a request for help seems like a rebuff. All Jesus did and said was to glorify God. He would not be glorified if men came to him just to see miracles. Jesus wanted all who came to him to be genuine about finding out if he was the Christ, not just to see signs. It made the man plead for him to heal his son before he died. Jesus told him he could go as his son would live. He took Jesus at his word and returned home.

Jesus is Lord of time and space

This man went to Jesus believing he must come to Capernaum to heal his son. After hearing his words, he believed Jesus had only to say the word to heal his son. On his way home, his servants met him and said his son had recovered at the exact time Jesus had said, *"Your son will live."* It made the man and his household believe. Jesus, the king of God's kingdom came to bring life – New Life, both then and today. In the life he gives, we live forever. Also it revealed Jesus' divinity and lordship over time and space, as the power of his word healed the boy at that moment even though he was twenty miles away. Jesus is the same today. As soon as he speaks, his word comes to pass. The power of his word to heal is not limited by time or space. If Jesus could heal that boy by not being physically present then he can heal each one of us today without being physically present.

The man did not do anything but believe Jesus. This is the way of grace that came in the person of Jesus. It is the way of faith – of believing not doing. This healing contrasts Law and faith. The Law always does and it is a life of stress. Faith always believes and it is a life of rest. The Law says we must do to please God. If we believe, we know He is pleased with us and we thank Him for His provision. If we believe, we will do, but it will be God, not us working in us.

Miracle 3

A miraculous catch of fish

'One day as Jesus was standing by the Lake of Gennesaret, with the people crowding around him and listening to the word of God, he saw at the water's edge two boats, left there by fishermen, who were washing their nets. He got into one of their boats, the one belonging to Simon, and asked him to put out a little from shore. He sat down and taught the people from the boat. When he had finished speaking, he told Simon, "Put out into deep water and let down the nets for a catch."

Simon answered, "Master, we've worked hard all night and haven't caught anything. But because you say so, I will let down the nets."

When they had done so, they caught such a large number of fish that their nets began to break. So they signalled their partners in the other boat to come and help them, and they came and filled both boats so full that they began to sink.

When Simon saw this, he fell at Jesus' knees and said, "Go away from me, Lord I am a sinful man!" For he and all his companions were astonished at the catch of fish they had taken, and so were James and John, the sons of Zebedee, Simon's partners.

Then Jesus said to Simon, "Don't be afraid; from now on you will catch men." So they pulled their boats up on shore, left everything and followed him.' – **Luke 5:1-11**

3. A miraculous catch of fish

Peter was a fisherman and had spent his life fishing on the Sea of Galilee. He would have known its waters well and known the best times and the best places to fish on the lake. However, on this occasion his knowledge did not prove fruitful as he had spent the night fishing and caught nothing. Next day as Peter was cleaning his nets, Jesus came along, got into his boat and asked him to put it out a little from the shore whilst he taught the crowd standing on the edge of the lake. When he had finished teaching them, he told Peter to put out into deep water and let down his nets for a catch.

The right time, the right place, and the right man

Luke places this event at the start of Jesus' Galilean ministry, after John the Baptist had been put in prison. According to Luke, this was the first time Jesus met Simon Peter. John 1:35-4:54 however, says he met Simon soon after his baptism and forty days of temptation. Then they went to a wedding in Cana in Galilee before attending the Feast of Passover in Jerusalem. After that feast ended, they spent time in the Judean countryside baptising alongside John the Baptist, before returning to Galilee and his ministry there began.

There were about eighteen months between their first meeting and this encounter on the lake. Peter would have seen enough of Jesus in that time to know that when he said something, it was best to do what he said. In Peter's mind, this was the wrong time and wrong place to catch fish and he probably was not the right person. Despite all this seasoned fisherman's experience and knowledge of fishing on the Sea of Galilee, he chose to obey Jesus' words. Because Jesus said it – Peter did it. When Peter obeyed his words, they caught such a large number of fish their nets began to break. They signalled to their friends in the other boat and they came and helped them. They filled both boats so full of fish their boats began to sink. At Jesus' words, they made the biggest catch of their lives. It was a net-breaking, boat-sinking catch of fish.

By listening to and obeying Jesus' word, Peter operated under the terms and conditions of the kingdom of God. In His kingdom it is always the right time. It is always the right place and it is always the right person. Jesus makes us the right person. Like Peter, we may not believe we are the right one or think we are worthy enough. We may think we are not experienced enough or not qualified enough.

However in Jesus' sight we are the right person. In his sight we are worthy enough and experienced enough and qualified enough. Jesus is the one who makes us worthy and it is he who qualifies us. Like Peter that day, there are times and there will be times when we must put aside our own knowledge and even our life experiences and accept that Jesus, the Son of God, who is God, knows better than we do. Jesus knows the beginning from the end and we can trust him to work for our good in every situation in life (Romans 8:28).

Obedience to Jesus' words

This miracle took place after Peter was obedient to Jesus' words, though all his instincts told him it was not the right time or the right place to catch fish. This miracle teaches us that when Jesus tells us to do something we must be obedient and do what he says, despite what we think or feel. We need to be obedient to his words even if we think we know better or our experiences in life have taught us differently. Peter's obedience resulted in abundance.

The abundance of the kingdom of God

When God calls us into his kingdom, he calls us into abundance. His kingdom is a kingdom of abundance; net-breaking, boat-sinking abundance. His abundance is not achieved by our own efforts. It is achieved by receiving His abundant supply – His supernatural, abundant supply. It was the abundance of God's supply that amazed Peter and the others. As experienced fishermen they knew that it was impossible to catch that quantity of fish in that place on the Sea of Galilee at that time of day. God will always provide far more than we could ask for or imagine (Ephesians 3:20).

God's goodness leads to repentance

After Peter saw the miracle catch of fish Jesus had provided, he fell at his feet in repentance and asked Jesus to go away from him because he was a sinful man. God's abundant provision of a net-breaking, boat-sinking catch of fish led to his repentance. His abundant goodness enabled Peter to see how sinful he was and that and that alone led him to repent. It was not that Peter's repentance led him into the abundance of God's goodness. And it is the same for us. We must learn what Peter learned that day. It is God's goodness that leads us to repentance (Romans 2:4). It is not our repentance that leads us to His goodness. Our good deeds, words and thoughts will never lead us into God's goodness. It is always God who takes the initiative. When our heavenly Father takes the initiative and shows us the abundance of His goodness and provision (His undeserved favour), we are humbled and repent. As it is God who takes the initiative, He gets the glory.

After Peter, Andrew, James and John experienced God's abundant goodness to them, despite their unworthiness, Jesus told them to leave everything and follow him. The four disciples obeyed and left everything and followed him. God deals with us in the same way today. When we experience His abundant goodness and see there is nothing in us to qualify us to receive the abundance of His grace in Christ, we too will leave everything and follow Jesus.

In his love for these disciples, Jesus let them get to know him for eighteen months before asking them to leave everything and follow him. During that time they had heard his teachings and witnessed his miracles and healings. After waiting eighteen months to call the disciples, Jesus would have known they had no doubt about what they were getting themselves into and who they were getting into it with. And Jesus does the same for us today. For some the call is immediate, but for the majority, Jesus lets us get to know him, his words and his ways before he asks us to leave everything and follow him.

It is easier to leave everything on a high

Jesus asked the disciples to leave everything after this miracle and not before. The experienced fishermen had spent all night fishing and caught nothing. If Jesus had called them after a night of failure they may not have believed they would succeed at fishing for men. If they could not catch fish, how could they catch men? Jesus is God, Creator of all things. When he provided a miraculous catch of fish, Jesus showed them he was the Creator and knew where the fish were in 'their lake'. If he could provide a huge catch in their area of expertise, then under his tuition they would excel in his area of expertise. Jesus knew where the men were who needed catching.

Also, it is easier to leave a way of life when we have reached the peak in our profession. If the disciples had dreamt of the day when they would make such a catch of fish that their nets would be full to breaking and that their boats would be full enough to sink, Jesus made that dream a reality that day. In the kingdom of God, when God fills our nets, it is always abundantly above all we could ask or imagine. God's supply always exceeds our demands. That night, the lake provided nothing for his disciples. However, with Jesus, their nets were filled to breaking and their boats to sinking. It is a wonderful demonstration of the abundance of the kingdom of God.

The call to ministry

This miracle teaches us about ministry. When we come to salvation and Jesus calls us, he calls us to ministry. God our heavenly Father has good works He has pre-ordained for us to do as we walk in His plan for our lives (Ephesians 2:10). In His loving grace, He gives us the gifts to do His work. It was the four fishermen's call to ministry and shows how God brings us into ministry. Often it begins with failure. They had fished all night and caught nothing. They were fishermen and had failed at what they were meant to do: catch fish. It was their calling in life and they were failing at it. In God's kingdom ministry begins after failure. It is when we realise we can do nothing without God.

In His grace, God shows us we can do nothing without Him, but often we learn this lesson the hard way – like Moses when he attempted to redeem Israel from slavery in Egypt in his own strength. He failed miserably when he killed an Egyptian and fled to Midian for forty years. By then, any thoughts of being Israel's redeemer had gone. After forty years God called him again to rescue Israel. Moses had tried and he had failed. First time he had tried and failed in his own ability, like Peter fishing on the lake. Then Moses went in obedience to God and through him, God redeemed Israel from Egypt.

Like Peter and Moses, we must realise we can do nothing without Jesus. Unless he is really working in us we will not achieve much. Without his power, anointing and leading we will do little. Peter had to learn he could not do things in his own strength but do them according to Jesus' will. Peter submitted to Jesus' instructions. If he had been doing it himself he would have given up. There was no logic to it. All his experience told him it was not the time to catch fish. Why would he do it all again after failing all night to catch anything? But, he had a fresh try at fishing at Jesus' word and in his presence. As a result, the miracle occurred and his nets were filled to bursting.

When Peter saw God had provided him with this miracle, he felt ashamed and sinful. He could not see how God could use a man as sinful as him and he told Jesus to go away. The good news is, Jesus took no notice and ignored his protests. He did not disagree he was sinful. Peter was telling the truth, but Jesus was still going to make him a, 'fisher of men'. Like Peter, we may feel unworthy of our calling, but Jesus knows everything about us. We are saved by grace and are ministered to by grace. He has a plan for us to take part in and takes no notice of how undeserving we think we are. God knew Peter was a coarse fisherman, who had been the worst of men, but it did not stop Him using him. Like Peter, our gifting is not based on how good or how holy we are. It is by grace and is based on Jesus' finished work on the cross. That is how and why God can use us and will use us, no matter how unworthy we think we are.

Miracle 4

Demoniac healed on a Sabbath

'They went to Capernaum and when the Sabbath came, Jesus went into the synagogue and began to teach. The people were amazed at his teaching for he taught them as one who had authority and not as the teachers of the law. Just then a man in their synagogue who was possessed by an evil spirit cried out, "What do you want with us, Jesus of Nazareth? Have you come to destroy us? I know who you are – the Holy One of God!"

"Be quiet!" said Jesus sternly. "Come out of him!" The evil spirit shook the man violently and came out of him with a shriek.

The people were all so amazed they asked each other, "What is this? A new teaching and with authority! He gives orders to evil spirits and they obey him and come out."' – **Mark 1:21-28**

'Then Jesus went down to Capernaum, a town in Galilee, and on the Sabbath began to teach the people. They were amazed at his teaching because his message had authority. In the synagogue, there was a demon-possessed man. He cried out at the top of his voice, "Ha! What do you want with us, Jesus of Nazareth? Have you come to destroy us? I know who you are – the Holy One of God!"

"Be quiet!" said Jesus sternly. "Come out of him!" The demon threw the man down and came out without injuring him. All the people were amazed and said, "What is this teaching? With authority and power he gives orders to evil spirits and they come out."' – **Luke 4:31-37**

4. Demoniac healed on a Sabbath

The healing of the demon-possessed man in the synagogue in Capernaum on the Sabbath is the first healing recorded in the Gospels of Mark and Luke. It is the first of seven healings Jesus performed on Sabbaths during his time of ministry:

Seven healings on the Sabbath
1. Healing of a demoniac in the synagogue (Mark 1:21-28)
2. Jesus healed Peter's mother-in-law (Mark 1:29-31)
3. Jesus healed a man's shrivelled hand (Mark 3:1-6)
4. Jesus healed a paralytic in Jerusalem (John 5:1-47)
5. Jesus healed a blind man in Jerusalem (John 9:1-41)
6. Jesus healed a crippled woman (Luke 13:10-21)
7. Jesus healed a man with dropsy (Luke 14:1-24)

Jesus' power over evil and the Devil

Mark 1:21-28 and Luke 4:31-37 say Jesus casting out an evil spirit in the synagogue in Capernaum was the first healing he performed. It demonstrated his power and authority over all the powers of evil. It confirmed the truth that the reason Jesus came was to destroy the works of the devil (1 John 3:8). To destroy them, Jesus first had to expose evil and the powers of evil, which was what he did that day in the synagogue. It made the evil spirit possessing the man cry out. It had no choice. Jesus' presence had exposed the power of evil.

We must never believe that the Devil is an equal match to God or that he is as powerful as God. Satan is a created being. God is not created. God created him. Jesus said that he saw Satan, *'fall like lightning from heaven.'* (Luke 10:18). Lightning travels at 300,000 kilometres per second. So God cast Satan out of heaven in an instant. That is how powerful God is. He is a million times more powerful than Satan and his forces of evil. Jesus came to destroy the Devil's works and he has the power to do it. One word from Jesus was enough to cast out the demon from the man in the synagogue in Capernaum.

Jesus is the Son of God and is God

The first time that Jesus was recognised as the Son of God during his time of ministry was by an evil spirit. A created being recognised its Creator had come to Earth as a man. However, that which was created had to obey its Creator. When Jesus said, "*Be quiet!*" it had to be quiet. When he said, "*Come out of him!*" It had to come out of him. Jesus was going to reveal his identity in his own timeframe and not let any evil power interrupt his schedule. That day, he showed his power and authority over evil spirits and all the powers of evil. Jesus had the power and authority then and he has it now.

The power in Jesus' words

Jesus' first four miracles all resulted from the words he spoke. In the synagogue in Capernaum, Jesus told the demon, "*Come out of him!*" and it came out of the man (Mark 1:25-26). In Peter's boat on the Sea of Galilee, he told his disciples, "*Put out into deep water, and let down your nets for a catch.*" When they did, they caught a miraculous catch of fish (Luke 5:4-7). In Cana, when Jesus told the royal official, "*You may go. Your son will live.*" His son, who was sick in Capernaum was healed at that exact time (John 4:50-53). At the wedding in Cana, when Jesus told the servants, "*Fill the jars with water*" and "*Draw some out and take it to the master of the banquet!*" the water turned into the best of wines (John 2:7-9).

These four miracles show the power and authority of Jesus' words. When Jesus speaks, what he says happens. Every word of God achieves the purpose for which He sends it (Isaiah 55:11). When God spoke, the universe came into existence. By God's word, the visible world was created from that which was invisible. He replaced that which was not with that which was and Jesus, God's Son continued to do this when he came as a man to minister on Earth. His word changed that which was not to that which was and that which was unseen to that which was seen: water to wine; sickness to health; empty nets to full nets; and evil oppression to freedom.

Obedience to Jesus' words

Jesus' first four miracles happened after he spoke and his words were obeyed. When Jesus told a demon *"Be quiet! Come out of him!"* it obeyed. It did not say another word and left the man (Mark 1:25-26). When Jesus told Peter: *"Put out into deep water and let down your nets for a catch,"* he obeyed and a miracle net-breaking, boat-sinking catch of fish occurred (Luke 5:4-7). After Jesus told the royal official in Cana, *"You may go. Your son will live,"* the man obeyed Jesus' words and returned home. On the way he was told that his son who was dying in Capernaum had recovered at the exact time Jesus had said, *"Your son will live"* (John 4:50-53). At the wedding in Cana, he told the servants, *"Fill the jars with water."* They obeyed and filled them with water. Then he said, *"Now draw some out and take it to the master of the banquet!"* They obeyed and when they served it to the master of the banquet, the water had turned into the best of wines (John 2:7-9).

These four miracles confirm the truth of his mother's words about Jesus at the wedding in Cana: *"Do whatever he tells you!"* (John 2:5). Peter on the Sea of Galilee; the servants at the wedding in Cana in Galilee; the royal official from Capernaum in Galilee all did what Jesus told them. Even the demon who was possessing the man in the synagogue in Capernaum obeyed him. When we believe and trust in Jesus and in his words and do what he says, we will experience the abundance of the kingdom of God. We will experience the New Wine of His kingdom. We will experience deliverance from all evil and from all the powers of evil. We will experience healing and health to our bodies and we will experience in our lives, the net-breaking, boat-sinking abundance of God's provision in Jesus Christ.

Miracle 5

Jesus healed Peter's mother-in-law

'When Jesus came into Peter's house, he saw Peter's mother-in-law lying in bed with a fever. He touched her hand and the fever left her. She got up and began to wait on him.' – **Matthew 8:14-15**

'As soon as they left the synagogue, they went with James and John to the home of Simon and Andrew. Simon's mother-in-law was in bed with a fever, and they told Jesus about her. So he went to her, took her by the hand and helped her up. The fever left her and she began to wait on them.' – **Mark 1:29-31**

'Jesus left the synagogue and went to the home of Simon. Now Simon's mother-in-law was in bed suffering from a high fever and they asked Jesus to help her. So Jesus went and bent over her and rebuked the fever, and it left her. <u>She got up at once</u> and began to wait on them.' – **Luke 4:38-39**

5. Jesus healed Peter's mother-in-law

After Jesus cast out the demon in the synagogue in Capernaum on the Sabbath, he went to the home of Andrew and Simon. There, they told him Peter's mother-in-law was ill. Jesus could have told his disciples not to worry as she would recover naturally or he could have told them to let her sleep it off as she would be fine in the morning. But he did not do that, for he is not like that. Jesus is full of love and compassion. He cares about every detail of our lives. If a loved one is unwell, he understands the pain of those who are sick and the pain of those who love and look after them. Jesus wants to be involved in all parts of our lives. He wants us to involve him when we or our loved ones are sick. He wants to help and bring his healing to us and to them.

The healing of Peter's mother-in-law shows us that Jesus wants us to tell him about our loved ones who are sick. He loves to involve us in his ministry. He wants us to bring our sick to him and bring him to our sick. Jesus loves to heal and is able and willing to heal. Jesus is healing. It is who he is. It is his character. God is glorified when we are healed by Jesus. He wants us to bring glory to God. We can do that by bringing our loved ones who are sick to Jesus (or by bringing them to him in Church) believing he is healing and is willing and able to heal all who come to him. Like Peter's mother-in-law, the only thing that qualifies us to receive Jesus' healing is to be sick.

Luke 4:39 says Jesus rebuked the fever in Peter's mother-in-law. The fact he rebuked the fever shows it was an evil entity that could hear and that it should not be in her. Sickness is not from God. It came to this world as a result of Adam's fall in the Garden of Eden. This healing shows the source of sickness is evil. 1 John 3:8 says, '*The reason the Son of God appeared was to destroy the devil's work.*' Jesus, who loved righteousness and hated wickedness could not bear to see evil hurting those he loved and not do anything about it. So he went to Peter's mother-in-law and rebuked the fever.

The moment it heard Jesus' word; the fever left her. Many today try to sweat out a fever, but evil cannot be sweated out. We cannot sweat out the Devil. He can stand all the heat we apply to him, but he cannot stand the word of God. He cannot stand against Jesus or Jesus' name. If we believe – our deliverance is assured, just as it was for Peter's mother-in-law when Jesus cast the fever from her that day. Jesus is just as ready to deliver souls today as he was then. When we receive Jesus as our Lord, the words of 1 John 4:4 are true for us: *'The one who is in you is greater than the one who is in the world.'* When we believe Jesus is the Son of God, who is God, he comes to live in us and is greater in us than all the powers of evil outside of us.

No one in his own human strength can meet the Devil. But anyone filled with the knowledge of Jesus and his presence and his power, is more than a match for the powers of evil. The Living Word is able to destroy satanic forces and all powers of evil. There is such power in Jesus' name. His name and faith in his name brings such power to bear against evil and sickness. Through Jesus' name the situation can be changed and a new order of things is brought into our lives. Jesus took on flesh that he might take upon himself the full burden of our sin and all the consequences of our sin, because on the cross of Calvary, God laid on him the iniquity of us all (Isaiah 53:6).

On the cross, the consequences of sin were dealt with once and for all. When Jesus said, "*It is finished!*" (John 19:30), his death destroyed him who had power over death (the Devil) and delivered all who were held subject to bondage through fear of death (Hebrews 2:14). His death brought deliverance from oppression and sickness for us all. We must learn to take his victory and shout in the face of the Devil: "*It is finished!*" We will not doubt, if we learn to shout this in faith. It is the power of the risen Christ we need. God has promised to pour out His Spirit on all flesh and His promises never fail. Our Christ is risen. Jesus died on the cross of Calvary for us to free us from all that mars and hinders us and to transform us by his grace to bring us out from under the power of the Devil into the glorious power of God, his heavenly Father.

When Jesus was brought to Peter's mother-in-law, he saw her lying in bed with a fever. He did not mollycoddle her or tell her she was ill because she had sinned and needed to repent before she could be healed. He spoke to the sickness itself. Jesus went for the jugular of what was causing everyone in that home pain – the fever. He rebuked it and it left (Luke 4:39). The fact he rebuked the fever shows it was not meant to be in her body. Sickness and disease were not part of God's original design for man. They came after Adam's fall. When Jesus came to Earth he brought God's kingdom. In it, sickness and disease must depart. As subjects of His kingdom, sickness and disease have no place in us. Jesus stood over Peter's mother-in-law who was laid down with a fever. He stands in authority today over every sickness and disease and over all the powers of evil. When Jesus rebuked the fever it had to leave her body. The created had to obey its Creator, Jesus Christ, the Son of God, who is God.

Jesus always raises us up

After rebuking the fever, Matthew 8:15 says Jesus touched her hand and the fever left. His first four miracles happened at Jesus' word. By his word, the evil power in Peter's mother-in-law's body was broken. Then he touched her, the fever left her and she was healed. He healed through the power of his word and the power of his touch. Jesus is the same today. His words have the same power now as they had then and his touch still has the same power today as it had then. All we need to do is believe and we will be healed.

His words and touch raised up Peter's mother-in-law. He is the one who raises us up from our sick beds and in life. He raises us up from a lowly position to the fullness of our height in God's kingdom. It shows the difference between life under the Law and life under grace. Jesus and his grace lift us up. The Law brings us down and condemns us to do to in order to receive God's goodness. Grace compels us to rest to receive God's goodness. Peter's mother-in-law did nothing to receive healing from Jesus. After he healed her, she could do what she could not do whilst she was sick – wait on him.

Miracle 6

Jesus healed all in Capernaum

'When evening came, many who were demon-possessed were brought to Jesus, and he drove out the spirits with a word and healed all the sick. This was to fulfil what was spoken through the prophet Isaiah: "He took up our infirmities and carried our diseases."' – **Matthew 8:16-17**

'That evening, after sunset, the people brought to Jesus all the sick and demon-possessed. The whole town gathered at the door, and Jesus healed many who had various diseases. He also drove out many demons, but he would not let the demons speak because they knew who he was.' – **Mark 1:32-34**

'When the sun was setting, the people brought to Jesus all who had various kinds of sicknesses and laying his hands on each one, he healed them. Moreover, demons came out of many people, shouting, "You are the son of God!" But he rebuked them and would not allow them to speak, because they knew he was the Christ.' – **Luke 4:40-41**

6. Jesus healed all in Capernaum

At sunset, all the residents of Capernaum brought all their sick and diseased and demon-possessed to Jesus at Andrew and Peter's house. Most of them would have been in the synagogue that morning and saw Jesus heal the demoniac (Mark 1:21-28). It seems that what they heard and saw caused them to believe he could heal their sick. However, they did not bring their sick to him to be healed immediately after the service in the synagogue. They waited until the Sabbath ended at sunset. Either they believed it was unlawful to heal on the Sabbath or that carrying the sick to Jesus was work, which was not lawful on the holy day (Leviticus 23:3).

Jesus' methods of healing

In the synagogue that day, it was a word from Jesus that drove the demon out of the man and it was a word from Jesus that drove the demons out of the possessed who were brought to him that night in Capernaum. It did not matter how many demoniacs were brought to Jesus; he gave the demons no quarter. He rebuked them and forbade them to speak. The created obeyed their Creator. When Jesus told them to go, they went. When he told them to be quiet, they were quiet. He was operating in God's timeframe. He was going to reveal himself to the children of Israel as the Christ, the Son of God who is God, in God's timeframe, not that of the Devil or his cohorts.

That night Jesus healed all the sick in Capernaum by laying hands on each one of them. It is the first time the Gospels record people being healed solely by Jesus' touch. So the Gospels reveal his first six healings were performed in four different ways, as shown below:

Jesus' methods of healing

1. With a word Jesus drove out demons
2. With a word Jesus healed the sick that were absent
3. With a word and a touch Jesus healed the sick
4. With the laying on of hands Jesus healed the sick

Jesus' variety of miracles

Jesus' first six miracles recorded in the Gospels were performed in a variety of ways: When he turned water into wine at a wedding in Cana (John 2:1-11) and when he provided Peter with a miraculous catch of fish on the Sea of Galilee (Luke 5:1-11), these were both **miracles of provision**. When he drove a demon out of a man in the synagogue on the Sabbath (Mark 1:21-28) and drove the evil spirits out of all the demon-possessed in Capernaum (Mark 1:32-34), these were both **miracles of deliverance**. When Jesus healed the royal official's son (John 4:46-54) and Peter's mother-in-law (Mark 1:29-31), these were both **miracles of healing**. In these six miracles Jesus revealed that he is Lord over nature; Lord over creation; Lord over the powers of evil and darkness; Lord over sicknesses and diseases; Lord over matter; and Lord over time and Lord over space. This is Jesus, the king of the kingdom of God. When we see Jesus as he is and when we see who he is, it increases our faith to come to him, believing that he has the power, the authority and the willingness to heal all our sicknesses and diseases and to deliver us from all oppression.

24 Hours in the life of Jesus

Mark 1:21-39 gives an insight into a day in the life of Jesus Christ as his ministry in Galilee began. Events took place over two days in one twenty-four hour period. On the first day, Jesus taught in the synagogue in Capernaum and healed a demoniac. Then he went to Peter's home and healed his mother-in-law. Jesus healed all the sick in town that evening by laying hands on them and he drove out all the demons with a word. He slept that night at Peter's home then next day, he went out early to pray. So, Mark gives a template of how Jesus operated each day as his ministry began. He would rise early to pray as communion with God his heavenly Father directed and equipped him for events that day. He would go to the synagogue to teach the people in that town and heal the sick that were there. Next, he would eat at someone's home and spend time with his disciples. If anyone brought their sick or oppressed to Jesus, he healed them all.

Jesus made Capernaum a sick-free town

From these healings, we learn that Jesus heals people any time of day or night or on any day, be it holy or not. Also it shows his driving out an evil spirit with a word was not a one-off event. He was not restricted to driving them out once. It was a continual driving out. The only reason Jesus stopped driving them out was because there were no more demons left in the people of Capernaum to drive out. Jesus' power to heal did not stop flowing. It was the flow of sick people in the town that ceased. Doctor Jesus' door is always open to all. He is always willing and able to heal all who come to him.

Events in Capernaum showed that Jesus could heal the demon-possessed with a word and the sick with a touch. By his word and touch, Capernaum became a sick-free zone. Jesus demonstrated his authority over demons and sicknesses. He was not restricted by locations. Jesus healed in the synagogue, in the home of his disciples and outdoors. Demons are created beings. They were created by God. The created had to obey its Creator. One word from Jesus was enough and the demons had to leave. They recognised his power and authority over them and submitted to it.

The residents in Capernaum witnessed Jesus' power and authority over sickness and evil spirits. They brought their sick to him to be healed and for their oppressed to be freed. We need to see Jesus' authority and power over all the forces of evil and demons and his power and authority over every sickness and every disease. We need to see the power and authority of Jesus' word and the power and authority of his touch to heal and to free all who come to him. We need to see and believe that Jesus is the same today as he was yesterday and will be tomorrow (Hebrews 13:8). Jesus' power and authority over sickness and oppression and all the powers of evil are still the same today as they were when he walked on planet Earth.

Miracle 7

Jesus healed a leper in Galilee

'A man with leprosy came and knelt before him and said, "Lord, if you are willing, you can make me clean!"

Jesus reached out his hand and touched the man, "I am willing," he said, "Be clean!" <u>Immediately</u> he was cured of his leprosy. Then Jesus said to him, "See you don't tell anyone. But go, show yourself to the priests and offer the gift Moses commanded, as a testimony to them."'
– Matthew 8:2-4

'A man with leprosy came and begged Jesus on his knees, "If you are willing, you can make me clean."

Filled with compassion, he reached out his hand and touched him, "I am willing" he said. "Be clean!" <u>Immediately</u> the leprosy left him and he was cured. Jesus sent him away at once with a strong warning, "See that you don't tell this to anyone. But go, show yourself to the priests and offer the sacrifices that Moses commanded for your cleansing, as a testimony to them."' **– Mark 1:40-44**

'While Jesus was in one of the towns, a man covered with leprosy came to him. He fell with his face to the ground and begged, "Lord, if you are willing, you can make me clean." He reached out his hand and touched him. "I am willing," he said. "Be clean!" <u>Immediately</u> the leprosy left him. Jesus ordered him, "Don't tell anyone, but go, show yourself to the priests and offer the sacrifices Moses commanded for your cleansing, as a testimony to them."' **– Luke 5:12-14**

7. Jesus healed a leper in Galilee

After healing the sick in Capernaum, Jesus went throughout all the towns of Galilee. Each day, he would have operated in the way he did that day in Capernaum (Mark 1:29-39). He would have begun the day in prayer with God. Then he would have taught in the local synagogue. Jesus would have healed all who came to him or were brought to him of every disease and sickness with a touch. He would have driven out all evil spirits from all the demon-possessed, with a word. He would have dined with his disciples and stayed overnight at the home of a local in each town where he stayed. This way of operating continued until Jesus healed a man covered with leprosy.

First healing in the Gospels

The healing of the leper (Matthew 8:1-4) is the first miracle recorded in the Gospels. The Holy Spirit through whom all Scripture is breathed inspired Matthew to record it as Jesus' first miracle. It did not happen first, but God wanted the first words on healing in the Gospels (spoken by a leper) to be, "**Lord if you are willing you can make me clean**." God's first words on healing were not about Jesus' power, authority, or ability to heal, but about his willingness to heal. The first thing He wants us to know about healing when we read His word and come to Jesus for healing is: He is willing to heal, no matter how bad the illness.

In Israel, the Law forbade lepers to be near other people. If a leper touched anyone that person became 'unclean'. If anyone touched a leper, the person became 'unclean' (Leviticus 13). The leper learned that Jesus had the power and authority to heal. He may have been told about it or saw others healed when Jesus laid his hands on them. According to the Law, this leper could not go to Jesus to be healed if he had to stay away from others. And he could not be cured if healing came by the laying on of hands as the Law forbade anyone to touch a leper. But whatever the Law said it did not deter this leper from coming to Jesus. It was what he had heard about him or had seen in him that made him determined to get to Jesus to be healed.

Leprosy and the Law

Humanly speaking there was no help for this man with leprosy as there was no cure for the disease. The Law had many rules about leprosy, but there is no record of any Jew being healed of it until Jesus and the kingdom of God came. This leper had not only heard or seen Jesus heal previously, but he knew he had such kindness and compassion, it made him approachable. So after he gave the Sermon on the Mount, the leper found a way to approach Jesus. Once he was in his presence, he was going to find out, once and for all if he was willing to heal him. He would find out if this man with the authority and power to heal would put his hands on someone like him who had such a contagious disease. The man covered with leprosy was not questioning Jesus' power or authority or ability to heal, he was questioning his willingness to heal someone as diseased as himself. That is why he said to Jesus, *"Lord if you are willing, you can make me clean".*

This wonderful healing of the leper is a parable to us. If leprosy is a visible picture of sin – our sin, then there is no earthly power that can deliver us from sin. Leprosy was a death sentence, and for us – sin is a death sentence. To escape death, we like the leper need to come to Jesus to be cleansed by him. This man was totally covered with leprosy (Luke 5:12). However, Leviticus 13:12-13 says if a man is totally covered with leprosy he is clean. Yes, if he is fully leprous, white with leprosy from head to foot, then he is clean.

In these Scriptures, God gives a visual image of us and our sin. If we come to Jesus and say we are only a little bit sinful then we are saying in leprosy terms, we are only a little bit leprous. Jesus will respond by healing our leprosy – that is the little bit we claim to have. If we come to him that way we will always struggle in our walk with him. We need to come to him and admit we are totally sinful. Then like a man who is totally leprous, he declares us totally clean. It is only when we admit we are totally sinful that we are able to receive his complete cleansing.

We must not trust in our own righteousness

If we say we are a bit sinful; we are claiming our self-righteousness has cleansed us of the rest of our sin. The more we claim of ourselves that does not need cleansing, the less Jesus' grace will be effective in our lives. Our self-righteousness and Jesus' grace are in direct opposition to each other. If we can cleanse ourselves, we do not need Jesus. If we cling to our own self-righteousness we will not experience the fullness of his redemption in our lives. Only when we come to him and admit we are totally sinful then will he declare us totally clean and his shed blood will have a hundred percent efficacy in our lives. This is true repentance. When we humble ourselves this way, Jesus' forgiveness, and healing are complete in our lives.

Nothing is too hard for Jesus and this leper knew it. The Law told him to stay away from people, but he found a way through the crowd to him. He believed and when faith lays hold, impossibilities must yield. When we touch the divine and believe God then our sins are forgiven; our sicknesses go and the circumstances in our lives change. Nothing could stop this man with leprosy whose heart was set on reaching Jesus. Today, no power can stop a sinner reaching him. If we have faith, we will not be denied. The leper knew Jesus could heal him, but he had to get close to him, for him to do it. He managed it and asked Jesus if he was willing to heal him. Was Jesus willing?

Jesus is willing to heal

Like the leper, we will find Jesus is willing – always more willing to work in our lives than we are to give him the opportunity to work in them. Our problem is, we do not come to him. We do not ask him for what he is more than willing to give. He is always willing to heal. He is the God who heals us. He is always willing to provide for us. He is the God who provides. He is always willing to feed us at all levels. He is the Bread of Life. He is always willing to help us. He is our Good Shepherd who cares for us, watches over us and wants the best for us and will use every situation in our lives for good.

Come to Jesus

Like the leper, we need to see Jesus' kindness and approachability. If we are definite when we come to Jesus Christ we will never go away disappointed. His life will flow into us and we will be delivered. It happened with the leper and each time he laid hands on the sick. Jesus is the same yesterday, today and forever (Hebrews 13:8). Today he says to us as he said to the leper, "I am willing – be cleansed!" Jesus has an overflowing cup for us. It is fullness of life. It is abundance. It is exhaustless. It does not matter how desperate our situation is, Jesus will meet us in our absolute helplessness. If we believe then all things are possible – nothing is impossible.

There are no add-ons. We do not have to input anything on our part, all we have to do is believe. God has a wonderful plan for us. It is a simple plan. His plan is: '**Come to Jesus!**' When we come to Jesus, we find he is the same today as he was in the days of the Gospel. Jesus still has authority and power to heal. And Jesus' answer to the question, "Will he heal me?" is the same answer he gave the leper almost two thousand years ago, "Yes I am willing!" He is willing and he is able. Let him make you clean. It does not matter how awful the sickness or disease is, Jesus will make you clean.

The clean makes the unclean clean

According to the Law, if a clean person touched an unclean person (this leper was unclean because of his leprosy) then the clean person would become unclean. But this was not any person touching the leper. It was Jesus, the Son of God, who is God. It was Jesus who brought God's kingdom to this Earth. In this kingdom, when the clean touches the unclean, it is the unclean who becomes clean. In the Law, the unclean makes a clean person unclean. In God's kingdom the clean makes the unclean clean. This is the beauty of the eternal God's grace He gives us in Jesus His Son. The consequences of it are the opposite to the consequences of the Law God gave through the man Moses.

Jesus' touch of compassion

The first thing Jesus did when this leper came to him for healing was to touch him. Jesus could have just said the word and the man would have been healed. However, he did not. He reached out and touched him. It is a wonderful demonstration of his compassion. The Gospels do not say how long the man had been a leper. The Law forbade him from touching anyone or from anyone touching him, so he would not have had any human contact since becoming leprous. In his compassion Jesus would have seen this and reached out and touched him. Then he healed him with a word. The word healed him of his leprosy, but the touch restored his human dignity. This is the beauty of Jesus. It is the greatness and abundance of the kingdom of God. God in Jesus does not just heal one part of us; he heals all of us, at every level. We must never question if we are worthy enough or holy enough or perfect enough to come to Jesus for healing. This account tells us Jesus receives us and heals us no matter how bad our condition is.

Jesus sent the leper to the priests

After Jesus had healed this man of his leprosy, he sent him to the priests to offer the gift that Moses had commanded as a testimony to them. This is the first time in the Bible that mention is made of a Hebrew being cured of leprosy and being sent to the priests to be pronounced clean. 2 Kings 5:1-27 does record the account of a man named Naaman being healed of leprosy in Israel by Elijah the prophet. However, he was not a Jew. He was the commander of the army of the king of Aram. He was healed when he obeyed Elijah's word to go and dip himself in the River Jordan seven times.

The provision for cleansing lepers and the duties the priests were to perform in order to cleanse the lepers were given to Moses by God during the Exodus, as recorded in Leviticus 14. Jesus' healing of this leper was God's testimony to the Jews, their priests and religious leaders that God's Messiah had come to redeem His people.

The cleansing process

When God instructed Moses about cleansing lepers in Leviticus 14, he said that when the man was healed of leprosy, he must bring two pigeons or doves to the priest and the priest would pronounce him clean and make atonement for him. He would kill one of the two birds then dip the other bird in its blood and sprinkle the leper seven times with the blood then pronounce him clean.

As seven is the number of perfection in the Bible, the sprinkled blood made the leper perfectly clean. After this, the priest would put blood on the man's right ear lobe and on the thumb of his right hand and on the big toe of his right foot. Then he would put some oil on the man's right ear lobe, on the thumb of his right hand and on the big toe of his right foot. Then he would put the remainder of the oil that was in his hand on the man's head (Leviticus 13:1-14:32).

The blood of animals shed for the atonement for sin is a 'type' or a forerunner of Jesus' blood that was shed on the cross of Calvary to atone for the sins of the world. The blood on the man's ear purified his hearing to hear and receive the truth. The blood on the thumb of his right hand meant that all he put his hand to would be pure. The blood on his right toe meant that everywhere he went, his steps would be true. In the same way, Jesus' shed blood on the cross purifies us from all of our sins, past, present and future.

The oil poured on the man's head symbolises the anointing of the Holy Spirit. Only three types of people were anointed with oil under the Old Covenant: kings, priests and prophets. When Jesus brought the kingdom of God to Earth, we see a leper, the most unclean of people being cleansed and receiving the same anointing that was bestowed on kings, priests and prophets. This is the Good News of the kingdom of God, where the lowest of the low are transformed to the highest of the high. No wonder the Holy Spirit ordained that this healing was the first one that was recorded in the Gospels.

Come to Jesus for healing

When Jesus turned water into wine, Mary came to him on behalf of the wedding hosts (John 2:1-11). A royal official from Capernaum came to Jesus on behalf of his sick son (John 4:43-53). Jesus' disciples came to him on behalf of Peter's mother-in-law who was sick (Mark 1:29-31). The people of Capernaum brought their sick and demonised to him to heal (Mark 1:32-34). This leper was the first to come to Jesus to get healing for himself. Today, this tells us, if we are sick, we must get ourselves to Jesus and ask him to heal us. Only Jesus heals. Doctors and medicines aid the healing process, but God alone heals. When He heals, He heals completely. His shed blood and death on the cross fully redeemed us from the curse of sin, sickness, disease and death.

There is nothing in ourselves that brings about or qualifies us for healing. It is all Jesus. It is all because of his finished work on the cross of Calvary. The death of His beloved Son on the cross was the price God set to pay for the sins of the world (every sin of every person who has been born or will be born). When he paid the price for us, he broke the power of the curse, sin, disease, sickness and death in our lives.

God alone set the price of our redemption. Out of His great love for us, He sent His Son to die for us. Out of His justice, He could not leave our sins unpunished, so He punished our sins in His Son, once and for all. As a result we go free and cannot be punished for our sins again. Jesus has already paid the penalty. In God's sight, Jesus' shed blood was the price He set to cleanse us from all our sins and free us from the curse of sickness, disease and death. God holds life and death in His hands. It is why we can come to Jesus for healing. Only Jesus heals. He is willing and able to heal all who come to him or who are brought to him.

Miracle 8

Jesus healed a paralytic

'Jesus stepped into a boat, crossed over and came to his own town. Some men brought a paralytic on a mat. When he saw their faith, he said to the paralytic, "Take heart, son; your sins are forgiven."

At this, some of the teachers of the law said to themselves, "This fellow is blaspheming!"

Knowing their thoughts, he said, "Why do you entertain evil thoughts in your hearts? Which is easier to say, 'Your sins are forgiven,' or to say, 'Get up and walk?' But so you may know that the Son of Man has authority on earth to forgive sins..." Then he said to the paralytic, "Get up, take your mat and go home." And the man got up and went home. When the crowd saw it, they were filled with awe; and praised God who had given such authority to men.' **– Matthew 9:1-8**

'A few days later, when Jesus again entered Capernaum, the people heard he had come home. So many gathered there was no room left, not even outside the door, and he preached the word to them. Some men came, bringing a paralytic, carried by the four of them. Since they could not get him to Jesus because of the crowd, they made an opening in the roof above Jesus and after digging through it, lowered the mat the paralysed man was lying on. When Jesus saw their faith, he said to the paralytic, "Son, your sins are forgiven."

Now some teachers of the law were sitting there thinking to themselves, "Why does this fellow talk like that? He's blaspheming! Who can forgive sins but God alone?"

Immediately Jesus knew in his spirit that this was what they were thinking in their hearts, and he said to them, "Why are you thinking these things? Which is easier: to say to this paralytic, 'Your sins are forgiven' or to say, 'Get up, take your mat and walk?' But that you may know the Son of Man has authority on earth to forgive sins..." He told the paralytic, "I tell you, get up, take your mat and go home!"

He got up, took his mat and walked out in full view of them all. This amazed everyone and they praised God, saying, "We have never seen anything like this."' **– Mark 2:1-12**

'One day as he was teaching, Pharisees and teachers of the law, who had come from every village of Galilee and from Judea and Jerusalem, were sitting there. <u>*The power of the Lord was present for him to heal the sick*</u>*. Some men came carrying a paralytic on a mat and tried to take him into the house to lay him before Jesus. When they could not find a way to do this because of the crowd, they went up on the roof and lowered him on his mat through the tiles into the middle of the crowd, right in front of Jesus. When he saw their faith he said, "Friend, your sins are forgiven!"*

The Pharisees and the teachers of the law began thinking to themselves, "Who is this fellow who speaks blasphemy? Who can forgive sins but God alone?"

Jesus knew what they were thinking and asked, "Why are you thinking these things in your hearts? Which is easier to say, 'Your sins are forgiven' or to say, 'Get up and walk'? But so you may know that the Son of Man has authority on earth to forgive sins..." He said to the paralysed man, "I tell you, get up, take your mat and go home!" Immediately he stood up in front of them, took what he had been lying on and went home praising God. Everyone was amazed and gave praise to God. They were filled with awe and said, "We have seen remarkable things today."' **– Luke 5:17-26**

8. Jesus healed a paralytic

The paralytic's friends would have heard or seen Jesus had authority and power to heal. Under the Law there was no hope or remedy for the paralytic in Israel. When Jesus brought God's kingdom to Israel there was hope. He is the only Jesus. He is the only life and the only help. Thank God, he triumphed to the uttermost on the cross. He came to seek and to save what was lost and he heals all who come to him. This man was helpless. He could not help himself get to Jesus. In response to the hope that is in Jesus, the men, with hearts full of compassion carried him to where Jesus was. The house was full. There was not even room by the door. It was crowded inside and outside. The men of faith were determined to get their friend to him at all costs. So they went on the roof and broke through it. Even if the way is blocked, with faith in Jesus there is always a way. Faith never fails. May the Holy Spirit give us a new touch of faith in God's power to have a living faith to trust him and say, "Lord I believe! Take us today and let us go through."

They lowered the paralytic through the hole in the roof right in front of Jesus. We need a faith like these men that will push through. We need a faith that will drop us right in front of Jesus. What a lovely place to drop into. When we drop in front of him; we drop out of our own self-righteousness; out of our own self-consciousness; and out of our unbelief. Jesus admired their faith. Faith that pushes through and overcomes obstacles is praised by God. Do we have that sort of faith? Will we do all that we can to get ourselves or our loved ones who are sick to Jesus to be healed? Will we allow obstacles to block us? It does not matter how we get ourselves or our loved ones to Jesus. What matters is, is that we get to Jesus. If others had not stirred us up or taken us to church, we would not have been saved. Many will not be healed unless we stir them up or get them to church. But we do not stir them up by condemning them. We stir them up by telling them about Jesus Christ, the Beloved Son of God – his abundant love, his great compassion and his willingness to heal and not condemn.

Faith comes by hearing

The men pressed through until their paralysed friend could hear Jesus' voice and liberty came to the captive. In the kingdom of God faith comes by hearing (Romans 10:17). People need to hear God's word about healing to have the faith to be healed. When Jesus saw the four men's faith, he told the paralytic, *"Your sins are forgiven!"* Why did Jesus say this to the paralytic? He did not need forgiving in order to be healed. However, out of his great love for this man, Jesus perceived that he needed to know he was forgiven to stop him condemning himself. Jesus did not tell him to repent in order to be healed. He forgave the man's sins to stop him condemning himself that he was paralysed because he had sinned. The abundance of Jesus' love and compassion flooded into this paralysed man and into his situation and he was able to receive his healing from the Son of God.

There is no condemnation in Jesus

Throughout the Gospels, there is no example where he condemned anyone for their sin who came to him for healing. Nor did he tell anyone they were sick because of their sin. Jesus even refused to condemn a woman caught in the act of adultery – yet the law stated she should be stoned to death (John 8:1-11). However, in some parts of the Church today people are told that they are sick because they have sin in their lives or they have not been healed because they have sin in their lives. Sometimes they are told they need to get themselves right with God before they can be healed or experience healing.

Thank God that Jesus is our template for life in his Church and in the kingdom of God and not man. If we were to take Jesus' mandate for healing and not man's then there would be a lot more healing in the Church today. If Jesus did not condemn people for their sin then neither should we or anyone in the Church condemn people for their sin. If Jesus did not tell anyone they were sick because of their sin, then we should not tell anyone they are sick because of their sin.

The religious leaders

The leaders reasoned in their hearts Jesus was blaspheming, as only God could forgive sins. They were right. Only God can forgive sins. But they could not see God in human form standing right in front of them. They based their judgments on reason, on their sense of reasoning. The Scriptures go on to say Jesus perceived in his Spirit what they were reasoning and addressed the issue. This healing challenges us about our attitude. If like the Jewish religious leaders, we rely on our own reasoning about Jesus, his works, his words, or even spiritual matters, we will come up short. We will draw the wrong conclusions. From those wrong conclusions we will make wrong decisions and we will live life incorrectly. If we follow Jesus' example and allow ourselves to be led by the perception of the Holy Spirit living in us, we will make the right decisions about the right things at the right time.

Which is easier to say?

Jesus asked the leaders if it was easier to say, *"Get up and walk or your sins are forgiven?"* It was easier to say, "His sins are forgiven" because no one could see if they had been forgiven or not, as the result would happen on the inside. It was harder to say, "Get up and walk!" Everyone could see if those words were effective by whether the man got up and walked or not. The man's need was to walk. Jesus forgave his sins. As soon as he received his forgiveness internally, his healing was demonstrated outwardly as he rose up. It will be the same for us – when we believe our sins are forgiven; we will walk out our healing. Inner forgiveness precedes the outer manifestation of the healing.

And the words in Psalm 103:2-3 will be fulfilled in us: *'God forgives all our sins and heals all our diseases'* as Jesus fulfilled them when he forgave and healed this paralytic. When he told him to get up, pick up his mat and go home, he was healed at once. By this healing, Jesus showed he had the power and authority to heal and to forgive sins, because he is God. God in human form had come to His people, but their leaders could not see it. They did not want to see it.

The power to heal

Jesus' first seven miracles occurred through the power of his word; the power of his touch; and the power of his word and touch. For his eighth miracle, the power of the Lord was present for him to heal (Luke 5:17). God's power was with Jesus to heal and by it this man became strong. He arose, took up his mat and went home praising God. We must not think about God on small lines. He spoke the word one day and made the world of things not seen. It is the kind of God we have. It is what Jesus did whilst he was here on Earth. He spoke the word and it came to pass. He spoke the word and demons fled. He spoke the word and sicknesses and diseases left.

God's word is so powerful it can transform lives. It is so powerful it brought this world into existence. The power in God's word makes the invisible visible. It is the power of His word. Psalm 107:20 says, *"He sent his word and healed them!"* And today His word has not lost its power. His word can bring things to pass today as it did in Bible times. By Jesus' word, this paralytic was cured. He healed him by telling him to do what he could not do, "Get up and walk!" It was the very thing the paralysis was stopping him from doing. Jesus' words spoke his healing into existence and he walked. He spoke what was not there into existence. He called that which was invisible (the man's healing) into being and that which was visible (his paralysis) into invisibility. Faith calls the things that are not as though they are (Hebrews 11:3). It is what Jesus did that day when he healed the paralytic.

Jesus is just the same today. He has not changed. There is none like him. God wants us to come near to Him and believe and claim His promises. They are, 'yes' and 'amen' to all who believe. Jesus is still setting the captives free today as he did in his days on Earth. We must believe that when we ask, we receive. It could not be otherwise. God said it, so it must be. May He reveal to us the greatness of His will concerning us. No one loves us like He does. May God give us such a touch of His reality today that we will trust Him all the way.

The right response

After the paralytic was healed by Jesus, he went home praising God. When the people in the house saw it they praised God as well and said they had never seen anything like it before. Something should happen every time we meet in Jesus' name so that people say, "We have never seen anything like this!" Whilst Jesus was on Earth, he always sought to glorify his heavenly Father. Everything he did and said was to glorify God. Jesus glorified his Father when he healed this paralytic and he glorified Him by all the miracles and healings he performed. He is still the same today. Jesus still wants to bring glory to his heavenly Father by healing all the sick who come to him or who are brought to him.

Jesus' blood was shed on the cross of Calvary for all men, for all time. His blood paid the price to meet all the world's needs and its cry of sorrow. He has met the needs of the broken-hearted and the sorrowful spirits. Jesus' sacrifice has met all the needs of every withered limb and every broken body. He has paid the debt for us all. He took up our infirmities and he bore our sicknesses and by his wounds we are healed. His word is Spirit and it is life. If only we will believe. When we believe, God's word will achieve its purpose in us.

Jesus restores us

It was only after Jesus had seen the faith of the four friends that he spoke to the paralytic. Have you ever questioned why? They in faith, got the man to where he needed to be – in front of Jesus. They let nothing stop them getting him to the one who could heal him. Jesus saw that faith in them. However, when Jesus saw the paralytic, he saw that he was not in the right place in himself to be healed. So the first thing Jesus did was to call him, "Son." Isn't Jesus beautiful? His words declared to those present, "I, the Son of God, proclaim you a son. I proclaim you; a paralytic are a son of Abraham. And as a son of Abraham you are also a son of God." So the first thing Jesus did was restore this man's status – how absolutely beautiful.

Our standing and status are in Jesus

Then Jesus declared, *"Your sins are forgiven!"* He declared the man sinless. In the sight of God he was sinless. Jesus proclaimed his status and his standing. He restored the man's standing before he could stand. Isn't Jesus lovely? He heals us on all levels. That is why he said what he said to the man. He needed his status and standing restored before he could receive his healing. After his friends put him in the right place to be healed, Jesus put him in the right place to receive healing by calling him son and by telling him his sins had been forgiven. He did not need his sins forgiven to be healed. He needed to know he was forgiven to be healed. He may have believed he was paralysed as a result of his sin. His illness would have stopped him attending the local synagogue and the feasts held in Jerusalem each year. It excluded him from religious life in Israel. It is why Jesus restored his standing and his status. He needed to know his status as a forgiven son in order to stop his wrong believing preventing him from receiving his healing.

Jesus proclaimed the man's status. He declared his standing then he healed him of his paralysis. He had to receive his standing in order to stand. When we hear Jesus' words – the words he speaks about our standing and our status – when we believe his words regarding our standing and our status – then we, like the paralytic receive our healing. Not only do we receive healing from Jesus, but we also receive all we are entitled to as children of God. We are washed and cleansed and are righteous in God's sight when we are in Christ. We are blessed and favoured and the curse of the Law is broken in our lives. All these are ours and so much more in Jesus, not because of anything we have done, but because of everything that Jesus did for us when he bled and died for us on the cross. His blood cleanses us from all our sins – past, present and future. He became our sinfulness so we could become his righteousness. He became our curse so that we could be blessed. All the blessings of Abraham come on us and all the curse of sin, sickness and death are broken. In Jesus we have healing and wholeness. What a great Saviour we have in Jesus our Lord.

When we look at our standing and status in Jesus Christ, the Son of God, who is God, all these benefits are ours. When we fix our eyes on Jesus – when we see him and see all that he did for us – when we see his finished work on the cross, like the paralytic our healing comes. It is how Jesus operated with the paralytic and it is how he operates with us today. He is unchanging. He is the same yesterday, today and forever. We must focus on Jesus and on our standing and status in him and not on our illness or circumstances. We must fix our eyes on the unseen and not on the seen. We do not stand in Christ because we deserve it, or earned it, or because of our good deeds, or anything else. We stand in him because he graciously gave us the faith to believe he is who he says he is. He will do the same for all who come to him.

Jesus spoke contrary to the man's condition

After Jesus restored the man's standing he told him to get up, pick up his mat and go home. In Jesus' eyes and in his thoughts the man could do all those things and by his words he did them. Jesus was talking kingdom language. Though the man was paralysed, Jesus saw him whole and he spoke to him as whole. He did not see him under the curse or Satan's dominion. Now this man was under the conditions of the kingdom of God, because the king of the kingdom was there. This paralytic was in the presence and the power and the authority of King Jesus Christ, the Lord of heaven and Earth.

Today, Jesus speaks to us as he spoke to the paralytic that day – contrary to our condition. He speaks to us as sons and daughters of God and as children of the kingdom of God even though we are humans. In God's kingdom there is healing and forgiveness. The kingdom of God is here. It came when Jesus came. The king of the kingdom is here to heal and to forgive. He has the authority to heal and forgive because he is the authority. Jesus is healing and he is forgiveness. He is the Lamb of God who takes away the sins of the world and by his stripes we are healed. As Jesus is the same today as he was yesterday and forever, he will heal and forgive us today.

Jesus condemned no one

Some people in life and unfortunately some people in the Church believe that God inflicts people with sickness because they have disobeyed Him or have sinned. This is why it is so important for us to know the word of God as recorded in the Bible. When we read the Gospels we see that Jesus did not bestow sickness on anyone whilst he was here on Earth, even though many of the people he encountered during his time of ministry were full of sin and evil. He did not refuse or condemn anyone who came to him for healing. If Jesus did not condemn anyone during the time he ministered on Earth then he will not condemn those who come to him for healing today. If he did not refuse anyone who came to him for healing when he was here on Earth then he will not refuse anyone who comes to him for healing today.

It is important to note that God is so pure, holy and true that there is no sickness in Him to give to anyone anyway. God is good and there is only good in Him. His goodness is best demonstrated in the fact that He sent His beloved Son, Jesus to die for our sins and the sins of the world on the cross of Calvary. When we see Jesus paying the price for our sins – when we experience his love, our hearts melt in admiration and God opens up all the treasures of the abundant, inexhaustible resources of the kingdom of heaven to us.

Miracle 9

Jesus healed a man's hand

'Going on from that place, he went into their synagogue and a man with a shrivelled hand was there. Looking for a reason to accuse Jesus, they asked him, "Is it lawful to heal on the Sabbath?"

He said to them, "If any of you has a sheep and it falls into a pit on the Sabbath, will you not take hold of the sheep and lift it out? How much more valuable is a man than a sheep! Therefore, it is lawful to do good on the Sabbath."

He said to the man, "Stretch out your hand." He stretched it out and it was fully restored, just as sound as the other. But the Pharisees went out and plotted how they might kill Jesus.' – **Matthew 12:9-14**

'Another time he went into the synagogue. A man with a shrivelled hand was there. Some were looking for a reason to accuse him, so they watched closely to see if he would heal on the Sabbath. He told the man with the shrivelled hand, "Stand up in front of everyone."

Then Jesus asked them, "Which is lawful on the Sabbath; to do good or to do evil, to save life or to kill?" But they remained silent.

He looked around at them in anger and, deeply distressed at their stubborn hearts, said to the man, "Stretch out your hand." He stretched it out, and his hand was completely restored. Then the Pharisees went out and began to plot with the Herodians how they might kill Jesus.' – **Mark 3:1-6**

'*On another Sabbath Jesus went into the synagogue and was teaching and a man was there whose right hand was shrivelled. The Pharisees and the teachers of the law were looking for a reason to accuse Jesus, so they watched him closely to see if he would heal on the Sabbath. But Jesus knew what they were thinking and said to the man with the shrivelled hand, "Get up and stand in front of everyone." So he got up and stood there.*

Then Jesus said to them, "I ask you, which is lawful on the Sabbath: to do good or to do evil, to save life or to destroy it?"

He looked around at them all, and then said to the man, "Stretch out your hand." He did so and his hand was completely restored. But they were furious and began to discuss with one another what they might do to Jesus.' – **Luke 6:6-11**

9. Jesus healed a man's hand

The account of the Sabbath healing of a man with a withered hand in the synagogue in Capernaum is recorded after the disciples ate grain on another Sabbath. Grain is only edible at harvest time. The barley harvest began after people returned home to Galilee from the Feast of Passover in Jerusalem in the first month of the Hebrew year. So at the start of Jesus' second year of ministry, the Jewish religious leaders were looking for a reason to accuse him. After just one year of preaching the good news of the kingdom of God and healing the sick, opposition against Jesus Christ had grown to the point where his enemies were looking for ways to kill him.

The sovereignty of God

However, nothing was going to thwart Jesus fulfilling the purpose for which his heavenly Father had sent him. 1 John 3:8 says, '*The reason the Son of God appeared was to destroy the works of the devil.*' It was the Devil who caused Adam and Eve to fall in the Garden of Eden. As a result of Satan's work, sin, disease, sickness and death came into the world. So when Jesus, the Son of God, who is God saw a man in the synagogue in Capernaum whose hand was shrivelled, he took action and told him to stand up in front of everyone.

This man did not come to Jesus and ask him for healing. Nor did anyone bring him to Jesus for healing. Jesus himself chose to heal him at that time and in that place. We must never forget Jesus is God and that God is sovereign. Yes, Jesus heals. Yes he is willing to heal and yes he heals all who come to him or who are brought to him for healing. But as God, he has the sovereign right to heal whoever he wants, to bless whoever he wants, to be merciful to whoever he wants and to favour whoever he wants, when he wants, where he wants and how he wants. This healing is a perfect example of the sovereignty of God at work. It was an opportunity for Jesus to show all who were present in the synagogue in Capernaum that day (and us) his divinity and to demonstrate life in the kingdom of God.

Finding rest in God

The good news of the Gospel of the kingdom of God is that through Jesus, all men and women can have peace with God now. That's right – peace with the all-powerful, all-knowing, all-seeing God. We can rest from our struggling and striving and trust in the love, protection and provision of our Heavenly Father. The fact he healed the man with a shrivelled hand on the Sabbath implies that he gave him his Sabbath rest. When Jesus healed him, he gave him rest from all his struggles – on the outside and on the inside. By grace, it is the rest God gives us in Jesus, His Son. It is a place where we receive rest from all our striving and struggling. We receive rest from trying to earn God's love and our salvation and healing. We receive rest from all our sicknesses and diseases. We receive rest from the death life – rest from the life under the Law that always demands us to do to please God in order to receive His Love, His salvation, His healing or anything else.

The Law hardens people's hearts

The religious leaders in the synagogue that day had no rest. They were constrained by the Law and would not be happy until they enforced it. Their eyes were fixed on Jesus to see if he would keep the Law. If he did not keep the Law, they were ready to punish him under the Law. So Jesus spoke to those under the Law with the Law. He asked them if it was lawful to do good and save life on the Sabbath or to do evil and kill. They remained silent. Jesus stared at them in anger, grieved by the hardness of their hearts. It was such a contrast to Jesus' own heart, which was so full of compassion and love for all men – even those leaders. And it is the same contrast that exists between grace and the Law. The hearts of the Jewish religious leaders were like the stone tablets that the Law – the Ten Commandments were written on. Jesus' heart was full of love, grace and mercy. Adhering to the Law filled the religious leaders' hearts with self-righteousness and it hardened them to the plight of their neighbour. Keeping the Law was more important to them than seeing their neighbour healed.

The religious leaders were holding to the code of the Law, but that day, Jesus fulfilled the heart of the Law when he healed the man with the shrivelled hand. Grace always gives and there is an abundant, inexhaustible supply. Law always demands. Those who preach the Law and those who follow it wear themselves out trying to keep its impossible demands. Only Jesus kept the Law and his death on the cross set us free from the Law of sin and death. We are no longer under Law, but under grace. The Law condemns, but there is no condemnation for those who are under grace.

As repentant sinners we receive God's forgiveness, healing, life and provision by believing in Jesus' finished work on the cross and not by trusting in our own efforts to keep the Law. All the righteous requirements of the Law are met in Jesus. When we believe and trust in him we are right in God's sight regarding the Law – not because of anything we have done, but because of what Jesus has done. When we see all that God has done for us in Jesus, we repent. We change our minds about God. We turn from sin and we trust fully in Him and in the death and resurrection of His Son Jesus Christ.

Jesus heals completely

Luke 6:6 says that it was the man's right hand that Jesus healed that day in the synagogue. Gospel writer Luke was a doctor. As a doctor, he would have made this point, because it is most likely it was the hand that the man worked with. So when Jesus healed this man's right hand, his healing was more than physical. Afterwards he would have been able to work. By healing his hand, Jesus restored his livelihood. He would have been able to earn a living and provide for his family. Rather than depending on them, now he could provide for them. This would have restored the man's dignity. This is the restorative life in the kingdom of God that Jesus brought when he came to this Earth. When Jesus heals, he does not heal only at a physical level – he heals at all levels. Jesus heals fully. Jesus is the same today as he was yesterday and he will be the same tomorrow. When Jesus Christ, the Son of God, who is God heals us today, he heals us completely.

Doing what he could not do

Jesus healed the man with the shrivelled hand by asking him to do what he was physically unable to do in his infirm condition – to stretch it out. As soon as he did what Jesus said, he was healed. Jesus spoke his healing into existence. He spoke what was not there into being. He called that which was invisible (the man's healing) into existence and that which was visible (his withered hand) into invisibility. *'Faith calls things that are not as though they are'* (Romans 4:17). His words have creative power. He did not live or operate on the lines of speculation. He spoke and it happened. In the beginning God spoke and the world came into being. Jesus speaks today and what he says comes to pass. Faith is the open door through which God comes. Jesus saves through the open door of faith and healing comes the same way.

Jesus' varied methods of healing

Jesus turned water to wine in Cana (John 2:1-11); and from Cana he healed a royal official's son who lay sick in Capernaum (John 4:43-53); he cast out a demon from a man in the synagogue (Mark 1:21-28); and healed all the demon-possessed in Capernaum (Mark 1:32-34) with a word. The Lord healed Peter's mother-in-law with a word and a touch (Mark 1:29-31). He healed all the sick in Capernaum (Luke 4:40) and a leper (Mark 1:40-44) by laying hands on them.

In the last two miracles we have looked at, Jesus healed people by asking them to do the very thing that their illness prevented them from doing: He told the paralytic to get up, pick up his mat and go home – the very thing his paralysis would not allow him to do (Mark 2:1-12). He told the man with the withered hand to stretch it out (Mark 6:1-6). It was something his infirmity would not allow him to do. Yet Jesus knew the power of his word to replace that which was visible (the man's paralysis and the man's withered hand) with what was invisible – their healing.

Miracle 10

Centurion's servant healed

'When Jesus had entered Capernaum, a centurion came to him, asking him for help. "Lord," he said, "my servant lies at home paralysed and in terrible suffering."

Jesus said to him, "I will go and heal him."

The centurion replied, "Lord, I do not deserve to have you come under my roof. But just say the word, and my servant will be healed. For I myself am a man under authority, with soldiers under me. I tell this one, 'Go!' and he goes; and that one, 'Come!' and he comes. I say to my servant, 'Do this!' and he does it."

When Jesus heard this, he was astonished and said to those following him, "I tell you the truth, I have not found anyone in Israel with such great faith. I say to you that many will come from the east and from the west and will take their places at the feast with Abraham, Isaac and Jacob in the kingdom of heaven. But the subjects of the kingdom will be thrown outside, into the darkness, where there will be weeping and gnashing of teeth."

Then Jesus said to the centurion, "Go! It will be done just as you believed it would." <u>And the centurion's servant was healed at that very hour</u>.' **– Matthew 8:5-13**

'When Jesus had finished saying all this in the hearing of the people, he entered Capernaum. There a centurion's servant, whom his master valued highly, was sick and about to die. The centurion heard of Jesus and sent some elders of the Jews to him, asking him to come and heal his servant.

When they came to Jesus, they pleaded earnestly with him, "This man deserves to have you do this, because he loves our nation and has built our synagogue." So Jesus went with them.

He was not far from the house when the centurion sent friends to say, "Lord, don't trouble yourself, I do not deserve to have you come under my roof. That is why I did not even consider myself worthy to come to you. But say the word and my servant will be healed. For I myself am a man under authority, with soldiers under me. I tell this one, 'Go!' and he goes; and that one, 'Come!' and he comes. I say to my servant, 'Do this!' and he does it."

When Jesus heard this, he was amazed at him, and turning to the crowd following him, he said, "I tell you, I have not found such great faith even in Israel." Then the men who had been sent returned to the house and found the servant well.' **– Luke 7:1-10**

10. Centurion's servant healed

The healing of the centurion's servant demonstrates the type of faith that Jesus wants those who come to him for healing to have. The servant was lying at home paralysed. The centurion loved him so much and was so keen to see him healed that he came looking for Jesus. This healing shows that when anyone seeks Jesus they will find him. There is no such thing as seeking him without finding him. Matthew 7:8 confirms that, *'whoever seeks finds.'*

Jesus' response to the centurion was so gracious, *"I will come and heal him!"* (Matthew 8:7). God sent His Son Jesus to his people, Israel. This centurion was a Roman, not a Jew, but when he asked Jesus to heal his servant, he willingly went with him. He is the same today as he was yesterday and will be tomorrow. He is always willing to come and heal. He still longs to help those who are sick today as he did during his time on Earth. He loves to heal people of their afflictions. Jesus is the same today as when he ministered in Israel. He still has power and authority to heal all sicknesses and diseases and to set the captives free.

Jesus was willing to go and heal the centurion's servant. However, the soldier stopped him from coming into his house. He told Jesus that he was not worthy to have him come under his roof. Then he told Jesus that all he had to do was say the word and his servant would be healed. The centurion went on to say that as a commanding officer in the Roman army, he knew what it was to give orders to those under him and to have his subordinates obey his orders. If he told his men, 'to go' – they went. If he told his men, 'to come' – they came. If he told his men, 'to do this' or, 'to do that' – they did this or they did that. When Jesus heard what the centurion said, he was delighted with the man's expression of faith and expressed his delight to those that were with him. Then Jesus told the centurion to go as his servant would be healed as he had believed. The army officer returned home to find that his servant was fully recovered, just as Jesus had said.

The secret of great faith

This event reveals another way in which Jesus healed people. It was the faith of the one who came to Jesus that brought about the healing. Of the twenty-seven healings that are recorded in the four Gospels, Jesus commended just two people for their, *'great faith'*: the centurion was one of them (Luke 7:9). Later we will see that a Syro-Phoenician woman who asked Jesus to heal her demonised daughter was the other (Matthew 15:28). We must look at what the pair had in common to warrant such praise from Jesus.

A centurion in the Roman army, who gave orders would have understood fully the execution of authority, but a mother would not. Interestingly, neither the centurion nor the mother was Jewish, so they would not have been under the Law. As they were not under Law, they did not disqualify themselves from Jesus' healing. The Law brings condemnation (Romans 4:15). As they were not under condemnation they had faith to see and believe Jesus had God-given authority to heal the sick and drive out demons. The Law is the opposite of faith and is not of faith (Galatians 3:12). It makes us work to receive from God. Grace enables us to receive freely from God. Those under the law cannot be expected to have faith.

The centurion and the mother were not under the Law. Free from the Law, they were able to believe and receive from Jesus. They came expecting him to heal (faith) and received what they asked for. The woman was not leaving until she had received her daughter's healing. It was great faith. The centurion saw clearly Jesus' God-given authority. He came to him relying on the practical execution of that authority to heal his paralysed servant and his great faith achieved the purpose for which it came. Throughout his ministry Jesus had shown his authority and power over sickness and demons. The centurion believed that all Jesus had to do to heal his servant was say the word. That was his level of faith and it brought praise from Jesus, who is God.

Jesus wants us to believe

It is the type of faith Jesus wants us to have. He wants us to believe in him and in the authority and power of his word. He wants us to believe what he says about our healing, as recorded in the Bible, will come to pass. When Jesus speaks a word of healing, the sick are healed. He wants us to believe he took up our diseases and carried our infirmities when he died in our place on the cross. He wants us to believe we are healed by his stripes (Isaiah 53:4-5). He wants us to believe he is the same today as he was yesterday and will be forever (Hebrews 13:8). Jesus has not changed and will not change. He was willing and able to heal all who came to him whilst he was here on Earth and he is willing and able to heal all who come to him today.

When we believe and trust in Jesus and his word, we too will be healed. Like the centurion's servant and the royal official's son, Jesus did not have to go and touch them physically in order to heal them. Jesus' healing power transcended both distance and time, because he is Lord of space and time. The centurion's servant and the royal official's son did not have to see Jesus in person to be healed. And it is the same for us today. We do not have to see him in person to be healed. Jesus' word was enough to heal then and his word is enough to heal us now. The most important thing is that we know Jesus and we know his word. When we do, we will have faith in Jesus Christ the Son of God, who is God and the power and authority of his word to be healed.

Neither the centurion with the paralysed servant nor the mother with the demon-possessed daughter doubted Jesus' words. At his word both of them returned home and both of them found the one they loved had fully recovered. Like the centurion and the mother, we must not doubt, but believe. We must take Jesus at his word. All his words are written in the Bible for us to read. They are true. And like the mother and the centurion, we must not doubt. It is in our trust and knowledge of the fact that God will never fail us or His word that we will be able to believe and receive our healing – no matter what our illness is.

Faith comes by hearing

Luke 7:3 says that the centurion heard of Jesus. Someone told him about Jesus. From what he had been told about Jesus – from what he had heard, he believed Jesus had the power and authority to heal his paralysed and dying servant by his word. Like this centurion, we need to believe all that we hear about Jesus that is written in the Bible. Like the centurion, we need to believe Jesus has the power and authority to heal. Like the centurion, we need to believe Jesus does not have to be present to heal us or the sick people we bring to him to be healed. We need to believe only in the power of Jesus, the power of his name, the power of his blood, the power of his word and his God-given authority to heal. The Gospel accounts reveals, the healing came about because the soldier heard about Jesus. This informs us that we need to tell people about Jesus. We need to tell people about his power, authority and willingness to heal the sick, the diseased and the oppressed.

Jesus raises us up

Jesus did great works because of his knowledge of the Father. Faith begets knowledge of God and fellowship and communion with God the Father, his Son Jesus Christ, and the Holy Spirit. Imperfect faith comes from imperfect knowledge of Jesus. Jesus said that the work of God was to believe in the one that He sent – that is to believe in Jesus Christ, His Son (John 6:29). We need to believe all Jesus said and did. We need to believe he took up our infirmities and carried our diseases and by his wounds we are healed (Isaiah 53:4-5).

Sickness and disease debilitate us. Jesus gives us life. Sickness and disease lays us low. Jesus lifts us high. He lifted Peter's mother-in-law off her sick bed (Mark 1:29-31). He raised up the royal official's son (John 4:43-53). He raised up the paralytic from his mat (Mark 2:1-12) and he raised up the centurion's paralysed servant (Luke 7:1-10). This is life in the kingdom of God. It is a life that raises people up. It gives them fullness of health and fullness of life in Christ Jesus.

Miracle 11

Jesus raised a widow's son

'*Soon afterwards, Jesus went to a town called Nain, and his disciples and a large crowd went along with him. As he approached the town gate, a dead person was being carried out – the only son of his mother, and she was a widow. And a large crowd from the town was with her. When he saw her, his heart went out to her and he said, "Don't cry."*

Then he went up and touched the coffin, and those carrying it stood still. He said, "Young man, I say to you, get up!" The dead man sat up and began to talk, and Jesus gave him back to his mother.

They were all filled with awe and praised God. "A great prophet has appeared among us," they said. "God has come to help his people." This news about Jesus spread throughout Judea and the surrounding country.' – **Luke 7:11-17**

11. Jesus raised a widow's son

This is the first account of Jesus raising someone from the dead. When he saw a funeral procession outside Nain, his attention was drawn to a weeping woman. She was a widow mourning the death of her only son. Jesus' heart went out to her. He approached her and told her not to cry. This is Jesus. He is full of compassion and demonstrated it at its highest level here. It is the account of a dead son being raised. However, it was not the dead that Jesus turned to first – it was the living. God is life. He is the God of the living. Firstly he gave his attention to the son's mother and comforted her. He was moved by her plight. Out of his great compassion Jesus understood and empathised with her grief. He gave himself fully to that before raising her son. There is such love and beauty in this simple action and his loving words, "Don't cry!" as he addressed her pain first.

It is a mistake to think God does not know what it is like to lose a loved one. No parent, grandparent, child, or lover has ever loved anyone as deeply or as completely as God loves Jesus. The Living God, Creator of the world; the all-seeing, all-knowing, all-powerful God, knows what it is to lose a son, to lose the love of His life. He knows the pain of separation by death. God in Jesus knows what it is to die. It was not an accident or by chance or a conspiracy of men that he died. God sent him to die in our place, for our sins. Jesus himself came to die for our sins so we could live. What love!

Death is the greatest pain in life. It is a destroyer. It devastates marriages, families, friendships and destroys people's joy. It robs people of their future and ends their hopes and dreams of a shared life for their loved ones. In ancient times if a husband died, his wife lost her main source of support. When this widow's only son died, she lost her only source of support. This healing shows Jesus' compassion is greater than death. He touched the coffin and those carrying it stood still. Jesus stopped death in its tracks. He told the young man, "*Get up!*" He spoke and death had to give the man up.

Life in the kingdom of God

This is Jesus. This is the kingdom of God. After Adam fell in Eden, the order of life was death. If Adam had not sinned, he would never have died. After the Fall, man was born, he lived then he died. It was the order of things. When the Law came, it enforced the death order. Failing to keep the Ten Commandments resulted in death – if you kill you die – if you commit adultery you die. Then Jesus came with the kingdom of God and a New Order. He brought life. When Jesus died and rose again, he defeated death. Death lost its power. In Jesus none die – all live. We will live and not die. We will fall asleep and wake in his presence, alive for ever. When we are in Christ, death and the fear of it are defeated and life is abundant.

When Jesus went to Nain, he brought God's kingdom to Nain. He brought the life of the kingdom into the widow's dead son. Luke recorded such beautiful words after Jesus raised her only son from the dead, "*He gave him back to his mother.*" (Luke 7:15). Oh how these words move us. Jesus is so lovely. He is so beautiful. Out of his great compassion for this mother, he raised her son to life then took him by the hand and gave him back to her. What a joyful reunion! What love! What a Saviour! Who could refuse him?

This woman was filled with grief and without support, because her son had died. Then Jesus came with his kingdom and restored her son to her. He restored two lives that day – hers and her son's. Like the son, we are dead until Jesus gives us life. We are dead to the things of God. Like the mother who lost her son, life without Jesus is full of pain. It is empty and lacks purpose. He came that we might have life to the full. It is what Jesus gives us. Where there was death, he gives life. Where there was loss he restores. Where there was pain he gives joy. Where there was emptiness, he brings fullness. This is Jesus our restorer. He restores that which was lost in our lives. He restores us from the emptiness of a death life to the fullness of eternal life. In this life all our needs are provided for in the kingdom of God.

Jesus brings abundant life

We receive all these wonderful things through Jesus. It is because he died for our sins on the cross of Calvary. It is because he loves us and oh how he loves us. The depths of his compassion and love are as striking as his power and authority over death. Jesus is all powerful and all loving. He is the Son of God. He is God in human form. He is the God of all compassion and abounding in love. Jesus demonstrated that compassion and abounding love when he raised the widow's only son from the dead in Nain.

John 10:10 says the Devil comes only to steal and kill and destroy; Jesus came that we may have life and have it more abundantly. Jesus is life and he gives us his life. He halted the process of death in this young man. Like that man, Jesus gives life to us, resurrection life. He raises us from death to life. Whether we would like to admit it or not the truth is, the life we were leading before Jesus came into our lives was a death life. All we had to look forward to was death. Spiritually we were as dead as the son in the coffin in Nain was physically dead.

However, when Jesus comes into our lives and touches our lives, we are born again. Just as he did that day at Nain, Jesus stops the funeral march in our lives and the journey of eternal life begins. He stops death in its tracks in our lives. Death is not the end anymore, because Jesus died and rose again victorious over death. The hopelessness and pain of death is replaced by the hope of eternal life in Christ. Just as he had compassion on the grieving mother, so Jesus has compassion on us. He has not changed. He is still full of love and compassion today and longs to pour his love and compassion into our lives – if we will let him. We need to repent. We need to change our minds to see him as the holy Son of God, who is God, who died for our sins on the cross and rose again. If we open our hearts, we receive his love and compassion and receive his healing and are filled with his abundant, eternal life.

Miracle 12

Jesus healed a blind mute

'They brought him a demon-possessed man who was blind and mute, and Jesus healed him, so he could both talk and see. All the people were amazed and said, "Could this be the Son of David?"

But when the Pharisees heard this, they said, "It is only by Beelzebub, the prince of demons that this fellow drives out demons."

Knowing their thoughts, Jesus said to them, "Every kingdom divided against itself will be ruined, and every city or household divided against itself will not stand. If Satan drives out Satan, he is divided against himself. How can his kingdom stand? If I drive out demons by Beelzebub, by whom do your people drive them out? So, they will be your judges. But if I drive out demons by the Spirit of God, then God's kingdom has come upon you. Or again, how can anyone enter a strong man's house and carry off his possessions unless he first ties up the strong man? Then he can rob his house.

He who is not with me is against me, and he who does not gather with me scatters. So I tell you, every sin and blasphemy will be forgiven men, but the blasphemy against the Spirit will not be forgiven. Anyone who speaks a word against the Son of Man will be forgiven, but anyone who speaks against the Holy Spirit will not be forgiven in this age or the age to come.

Make a tree good and its fruit will be good, or make a tree bad and its fruit will be bad, for a tree is recognised by its fruit.

You brood of vipers, how can you who are evil say anything good? For out of the overflow of the heart the mouth speaks. The good man brings good things out of the good stored up in him, and the evil man brings evil things out of the evil stored up in him. But I tell you that men will have to give account on Judgment Day for every careless word they have spoken. For by your words you will be acquitted and by your words you will be condemned.' **– Matthew 12:22-37**

'*The teachers of the law from Jerusalem said, "He is possessed by Beelzebub! By the prince of demons he is driving out demons." So he spoke to them in parables; "How can Satan drive out Satan? If a kingdom is divided against itself, that kingdom cannot stand. If a house is divided against itself, that house cannot stand. And if Satan opposes himself and is divided, he cannot stand, his end has come. In fact no one can enter a strong man's house and carry off his things unless he first ties up the strong man. Then he can rob his house. I tell you the truth, all the sins and blasphemies of men will be forgiven them. But whoever blasphemes against the Holy Spirit will never be forgiven; he is guilty of an eternal sin." He said this because they were saying, "He has an evil spirit."'* **– Mark 3:22-30**

'*Jesus was driving out a demon that was mute. When the demon left, the man who had been mute spoke and the crowd was amazed. But some of them said, "By Beelzebub, the prince of demons, he is driving out demons." Others asked for a sign. Jesus knew their thoughts and said, "A kingdom divided against itself will fall, and a house divided against itself will fall. If Satan is divided against himself how can his kingdom stand? I say this because you claim I drive out demons by Beelzebub. If I drive out demons by Beelzebub, by whom do your followers drive them out? So then, they will be your judges. But if I drive out demons by the finger of God, His kingdom has come to you. When a strong man, fully armed guards his house, his things are safe until someone stronger attacks and overpowers him and takes away the armour in which he trusted and divides up his spoils. He who is not with me is against me."'* **– Luke 11:14-23**

12. Jesus healed a blind mute

Matthew and Mark record this healing of a demonised blind mute before Jesus taught the crowd in parables by the Sea of Galilee in his second year of ministry. Luke recorded it in Jesus' final year of ministry with other events to stress the truths he was making in that part of his Gospel. All three writers focus on the response of those who saw the healing, rather than the healing itself, where a blind mute was healed after Jesus showed his authority and power over evil by casting a demon out of the man. The people were amazed and asked if Jesus could be the Messiah. When the religious leaders heard this, they condemned Jesus and declared that he drove out demons by the Devil. The crowd that day used their God-given voices to praise God. The Jewish leaders used their God-given voices to condemn Jesus. Like the crowd and the leaders, God has given us a voice to either praise Jesus or condemn him. God has given us the freedom to choose.

Blind to the truth

When the crowd saw Jesus in the right light they asked the right questions. The Jewish religious leaders were blind to the fact that Jesus was the Messiah, the Son of God, who was God. They were blind to the fact that the living, eternal God had come to Earth in human form and was standing right in front of them. The leaders were as blind spiritually as the man who had been healed was blind physically. They were blind to the truths of Jesus, their Christ and of God's kingdom.

They were spiritually dumb too, as their words bore no truth about the reality of God, His Messiah, His kingdom and His Son. Like them, before we know Jesus, we think we know everything about God, His Son, His kingdom and His word. The truth is we know nothing at all about any of it. Regarding spiritual truths we too are spiritually as blind as this man was physically blind. And the words we speak regarding God, His kingdom, His Son and eternal life reveal how little we know.

Bring the sick to Jesus

Like the people of Capernaum who brought all their sick and demon-possessed to Jesus (Mark 1:32-34) and the four men who brought their paralysed friend on a mat to Jesus (Mark 2:1-12), these people brought this blind, mute demon-possessed man to Jesus. Like the paralytic and all the sick and demon-possessed in Capernaum, Jesus, the Son of God, who is God, in his great love and compassion healed him.

This shows that part of Jesus' ministry consisted of him healing all who were brought to him. It reveals to us that we should bring all our loved ones, our neighbours, our colleagues, our classmates and all those we encounter in life who are sick to Jesus to be healed. Jesus is the same today as he was when he ministered in Israel, which means that when we bring our sick to him, he will heal them.

Miracle 13

Jesus calmed a storm

'Then Jesus got into the boat and his disciples followed him. Without warning a furious storm came up on the lake, so that the waves swept over the boat. But Jesus was sleeping. The disciples went and woke him, saying, "Lord, save us! We're going to drown!"

Jesus replied, "You of little faith, why are you so afraid?" He got up and rebuked the winds and the waves, and it was completely calm.

The men were amazed and asked, "What kind of man is this? Even the winds and the waves obey him?"' **– Matthew 8:23-27**

'That day, when evening came, Jesus said to his disciples, "Let's go over to the other side." Leaving the crowd behind, they took him along, just as he was, in the boat. There were other boats with him. A furious squall came up and the waves broke over the boat, so it was nearly swamped. Jesus was in the stern, sleeping on a cushion. They woke him and said, "Teacher, don't you care if we drown?"

He got up, rebuked the wind and said to the waves, "Quiet! Be still!" Then the wind died down and it was completely calm.

He asked them, "Why are you so afraid? Do you still have no faith?"

They were terrified and asked each other, "Who is this? Even the wind and the waves obey him!"' **– Mark 4:35-41**

'One day Jesus said to his disciples, "Let's go over to the other side of the lake." They got into a boat and set out. As they sailed, he fell asleep. A squall came down on the lake, so that the boat was swamped and they were in great danger.

The disciples went to Jesus and woke him saying, "Master, Master, we're going to drown!"

Jesus got up and rebuked the wind and the raging waters; the storm subsided, and all was calm. "Where is your faith?" he asked them.

In fear and amazement the disciples asked one another, "Who is this? He commands even the winds and the water, and they obey him."'
– Luke 8:22-25

13. Jesus calmed a storm

Jesus said to his disciples, *"Let's go over to the other side of the lake."* A storm arose and swamped the boat with water. They were terrified and thought they were going to drown. They woke Jesus who was asleep on a cushion in the stern of the boat and asked him if he cared or not if they drowned. Jesus got up and rebuked the wind and the waves. At his rebuke, they became still.

Like Jesus and his disciples on the lake, a storm can come up for us at any time in our lives. And like them it can threaten to drag us under. The disciples cried out to Jesus for help and he rebuked them for their lack of faith. If Jesus is in our boat in life and if he can sleep on a cushion in the stern, it says, no matter what storm comes up it will not drown us. We may get splashed and we may get wet, but we will not drown. So our first goal is to get Jesus into our boat.

If Jesus can be unaffected by a sudden storm rising up then so can we. It is worth noting Jesus said to his disciples, *"Let us cross to the other side of the lake"* (Luke 8:22). The fact Jesus said it meant they would get there. This storm in his life did not unsettle him and storms in our lives will not unsettle us if we fix our eyes on Jesus and trust what he says. We must not let circumstances or the storms of life drag us under. The disciples had their eyes on the storm not on Jesus or his words or they would have had the faith to believe they would arrive safely on the other side of the lake, despite the storm.

This shows us to trust what Jesus says and not doubt. Then we will be able to stay calm, no matter what life throws at us and sleep peacefully through the fiercest storm. We need to trust what Jesus says will happen. He rebuked his disciples' lack of faith when they asked if he cared if they drowned and for doubting they would reach the other side of the lake. Because of Jesus' selfless, sacrifice for us on the cross of Calvary, unlike the disciples we need never doubt if he cares enough about us or the situations in our lives.

Trusting our standing, not our circumstances

We need to believe what Jesus says and what his words say about our standing in him. If we are not secure in our standing in Christ then the circumstances in our lives will always affect us. We must never base our status in life on our circumstances. We must always base our status on our standing in Christ Jesus then the winds and storms that arise in life will never overwhelm us.

Once again, Jesus showed his authority and power over creation. The wind and the waves are part of creation and they had to obey their Creator, Jesus. When he told the wind, *"Be quiet!"* it had to be quiet. When he told the waves; *"Be still!"* they had to be still. At his rebuke the wind and waves died down. The disciples were amazed that even the wind and the waves obeyed him. They had seen demons obey him. They had seen fevers and sicknesses obey him. Now they had seen nature obey him. In regard to his identity, they had clearly forgotten the words of Psalm 107:29-30:

'*He stilled the storm to a whisper; the waves of the sea were hushed. They were glad when it grew calm and he guided them to their desired haven.*'

Miracle 14

Jesus healed two demoniacs

'When he arrived at the other side in the region of the Gadarenes, two demon-possessed men coming from the tombs met him. They were so violent that no one could pass that way. "What do you want with us, Son of God?" they shouted. "Have you come here to torture us before the appointed time?"

Some distance away a large herd of pigs was feeding. The demons begged Jesus, "If you drive us out, send us into the herd of pigs."

He said to them, "Go!" So they came out and went into the pigs and the whole herd rushed down the steep bank into the lake and died in the water. Those tending the pigs ran into the town and reported all this, including what had happened to the two demon-possessed men. The whole town went out to meet Jesus. When they saw him, they pleaded with him to leave their region.' – **Matthew 8:28-34**

'They went across the lake to the region of the Gerasenes. When Jesus got out of the boat, a man with an evil spirit came from the tombs to meet him. This man lived in the tombs, and no one could bind him anymore, not even with a chain. He had often been chained hand and foot but tore them apart and broke the irons on his feet. No one was strong enough to subdue him. Night and day among the tombs and in the hills he cried out and cut himself with stones. When he saw Jesus from a distance, he ran and fell on his knees in front of him. He shouted at the top of his voice, "What do you want with me, Jesus, Son of the Most High God? Swear to God that you won't torture me!"

For Jesus had said to him, "Come out of this man, you evil spirit!" Then Jesus asked him, "What is your name?"

"My name is Legion," he replied, "for we are many." And he begged Jesus again and again not to send them out of the area.

A large herd of pigs was feeding on the nearby hillside. The demons begged Jesus, "Send us among the pigs; allow us to go into them." He gave them permission and the evil spirits came out and went into the pigs. The herd, about two thousand in number, rushed down the steep bank into the lake and were drowned.

Those tending the pigs ran off and reported this in the town and countryside, and the people went out to see what had happened. When they came to Jesus, they saw the man who had been possessed by the legion of demons, sitting there, dressed and in his right mind; and they were afraid. Those who had seen it told the people what had happened to the demon-possessed man – and told about the pigs as well. Then the people began to plead with Jesus to leave their region.

As Jesus got into the boat, the man who had been demon-possessed begged to go with him. He did not let him, but said, "Go home to your family and tell them how much God has done for you, and how he has had mercy on you." He went away and told in the Decapolis how much Jesus had done for him, and everyone was amazed.' **– Mark 5:1-20**

'*They sailed to the region of the Gerasenes, across the lake from Galilee. When Jesus stepped ashore, he was met by a demoniac from the town. For a long time he had not worn clothes or lived in a house, but had lived in the tombs. When he saw Jesus, he fell at his feet and cried out at the top of his voice, "What do you want with me, Jesus, Son of the Most High God? I beg you, don't torture me!" For he had ordered the evil spirit to come out of him. Many times it had seized him, though he was chained hand and foot and kept under guard, he had broken his chains and been driven by the demon into solitary places.*

Jesus asked him, "What is your name?"

"Legion," he replied, because many demons had gone into him. And they begged him repeatedly, not to order them to go into the Abyss.

A large herd of pigs was feeding there on the hillside. The demons begged him to let them go into them, and he gave them permission. When the demons came out of the man, they went into the pigs, and the herd rushed down the bank into the lake and was drowned.

When those tending the pigs saw what had happened, they ran off and reported this in the town and countryside, and the people went out to see what had occurred. When they came to Jesus, they found the man from whom the demons had gone out, sitting at Jesus' feet, dressed and in his right mind; and they were afraid. Those who had seen it told how the demoniac had been cured. Then all the people of the region of the Gerasenes asked Jesus to leave them, because they were overcome with fear. So he got into the boat and left.

The man from whom the demons had gone out begged to go with him, but Jesus sent him away saying, "Return home and tell how much God has done for you." So the man went and told all over town how much Jesus had done for him.' **– Luke 8:26-39**

14. Jesus healed two demoniacs

After Jesus had calmed the storm, the boat arrived in the region of the Gerasenes. As he got out of the boat two demon-possessed men ran up to him and fell at his feet. Immediately the demons in the men recognised God in human form, calling him, 'Jesus, Son of the Most High God'. One of the men was possessed by a legion of demons. He begged Jesus repeatedly not to send them into the Abyss. These evil spirits were terrified about being sent to hell and pleaded with Jesus to send them into a herd of pigs that were nearby.

There are two things we can learn from the dialogue between Jesus and the demons. The first thing is that we should never make the mistake of believing that there is no such place as Hell. During his time on Earth, Jesus spoke about Hell to his disciples, to the crowds that gathered around him and to the Jewish religious leaders of his day. In all the times he spoke about Hell not one person challenged him about it or said, "Hell does not exist." The second thing we learn is the fact that Hell is so horrible that even demons and the powers of evil do not want to go there. If they do not want to go there, how much more then should we dread going there? Thank God, through His Son, Jesus, He has made a way for us not to go there, but to spend eternity with Him.

Instead of sending the demons into the abyss, with a word, Jesus drove them out into a herd of pigs. The pigs ran down the hill into the lake and drowned. It shows the words in John 10:10 are true: '*The thief comes only to steal, to kill and to destroy.*' The thief is the Devil and all the forces of evil. They came into the men and stole their peace of mind and their health and destroyed their families and their livelihood. If Jesus had not brought his kingdom into the two men's lives, the demons would have killed them. When they did not satisfy that desire in the two men, they went into the herd of pigs and killed all of them. Make no mistake, evil and Hell are realities and so is our victory over them in Christ Jesus, our crucified and risen Saviour.

Jesus reigns over all the powers of evil

One word from Jesus was enough to cast the legion of demons out of the man. If a legion was a group of a thousand soldiers in the Roman army then there were a thousand demons in this man. One word was enough to cast them out then and it is enough today. It did not matter if it was one demon or a thousand, at Jesus' word they had to go. It is the power and authority of his word and this is one of seven times Jesus cast out demons by his power and authority:

Demoniacs healed by Jesus during his ministry
1. Demoniac healed in Capernaum (Mark 1:21-28)
2. Demon-possessed blind mute healed (Mark 3:22-30)
3. Two demoniacs healed in the Gerasenes (Mark 5:1-20)
4. Demon-possessed mute healed (Matthew 9:32-34)
5. Seven demons driven out of Mary Magdalene (Luke 8:2)
6. Demonised daughter healed in Tyre (Mark 7:24-30)
7. Demonised son healed (Mark 9:14-29)

Seven is the number of perfection in the Bible. The Gospels record Jesus cast out evil spirits seven times to show he has perfect power and authority over all the powers of evil and the Devil. His power is a million times greater than all the powers of the Devil and evil. He had total power and authority over evil spirits then and he has it now. As his children we must believe and trust in his power and authority over all the powers of evil. We must believe and trust in the power of Jesus' name and his word. He has given all who believe he is Christ, the same power and authority over all the powers of the Devil and evil.

The evil spirits in the men were created beings and recognised their Creator who had come in the flesh. But evil could not stand in the presence of the pure and holy Son of God. The demons bowed down before their maker when the men they were possessing fell at Jesus' feet. As part of creation, they obeyed their Creator. When he said, "Go!" all these demons had to leave the poor men they were possessing.

The perfect place in life

Despite having a thousand demons inside him, the man was not so possessed that he could not run to Jesus to be healed. If he could do so, then we have no excuse for not coming to him to be healed. However, when the people in that region came and saw the man who had been demon-possessed sitting at Jesus' feet, dressed and in his right mind they were afraid. That is sad because being dressed and sitting at Jesus' feet in our right minds listening to his words is the perfect position that a believer can take in life.

The demon-possessed man was restored from nakedness, crying out and cutting himself to the perfect position in life. Jesus delivered him from his bondage and from a life of harming himself. Today, people who cut themselves need delivering. Jesus came that we may have life and have it more abundantly. There is no abundance in life when a person harms himself or others. The perfect place in life is to be seated at Jesus' feet, clothed and not naked in carnality and sin, but in his righteousness. Then we will no longer be at the whims of our carnal desires. The perfect place in life is to be in our right minds, which are open to Jesus' truths and open to his teaching, guidance, love, grace and the abundant provision of the kingdom of God.

Miracle 15

Jesus healed a bleeding woman

'While he was saying this, a ruler knelt before him and said, "My daughter has just died. But come and put your hand on her, and she will live." Jesus got up and went with him, and so did his disciples.

Just then a woman who had been subject to bleeding for twelve years came up behind him and touched the edge of his cloak. She said to herself, "If I only touch his cloak, I will be healed." Jesus turned and saw her, "Take heart, daughter," he said, "your faith has healed you." And the woman was healed from that moment.' – **Matthew 9:18-22**

'When Jesus had again crossed over by boat to the other side of the lake, a large crowd gathered around him while he was by the lake. Then one of the synagogue rulers; named Jairus came there. Seeing Jesus, he fell at his feet and pleaded earnestly with him, "My little daughter is dying. Please come and put your hands on her so that she will be healed and live." So Jesus went with him.

A large crowd followed and pressed around him. A woman was there who had been subject to bleeding for twelve years. She had suffered greatly under the care of many doctors and had spent all she had, yet instead of getting better she grew worse. When she heard about Jesus, she came up behind him in the crowd and touched his cloak, because she thought, "If I just touch his clothes, I will be healed." Immediately her bleeding stopped and she felt in her body she was freed from her suffering. At once Jesus realised power had gone out from him. He turned around and asked, "Who touched my clothes?"

"You see the people crowding against you," his disciples said, "yet you can ask, 'Who touched me?'"

But Jesus kept looking around to see who had done it. Then the woman, knowing what had happened to her came and fell at his feet, and trembling with fear told him the whole truth. He said to her, "Daughter your faith has healed you. Go in peace and be freed from your suffering."' **– Mark 5:21-34**

'Now when Jesus returned, a crowd welcomed him, for they were all expecting him. A man named Jairus, a ruler of the synagogue came and fell at Jesus' feet, pleading with him to come to his house because his only daughter, a girl of about twelve years, was dying.

As he was on his way, the crowds almost crushed him. A woman was there who had been subject to bleeding for twelve years, but no one could heal her. She came up behind him and touched the edge of his cloak, and immediately her bleeding stopped.

"Who touched me?" Jesus asked.

When they all denied it, Peter said, "Master, the people are crowding and pressing against you."

However, Jesus said, "Someone touched me; I know that power has gone out from me."

Then the woman, seeing that she could not go unnoticed, came trembling and fell at his feet. In the presence of all the people, she told why she had touched him and how she had been instantly healed. Then he said to her, "Daughter, your faith has healed you. Go in peace."' **– Luke 8:40-48**

15. Jesus healed a bleeding woman
The clean makes the unclean, clean

After healing the demoniacs in the Gerasenes, Jesus crossed the lake to Capernaum. A crowd gathered around him as he made his way to heal the daughter of the synagogue ruler. A woman who had bled for twelve years touched his cloak to be healed. When she did, he felt power leave him and asked who had touched him. When the woman came and explained why she had done it, he commended her faith. She believed Jesus was so full of healing virtue it overflowed from him and all she had to do to be healed was touch the edge of his cloak.

The Jewish Law said it was unlawful for her to touch the crowd or Jesus or his clothes. Leviticus 15:25-27 says when a woman had a continual flow of blood, it made her unclean. It was unlawful for an unclean person to touch anyone or anything that was clean. If they did the clean person or the clean object became unclean (Numbers 19:22). The woman believed that she only had to touch the edge of Jesus' cloak to be healed, but she would have to break the Law to do it.

Instead of expecting punishment from the Law she expected healing from Jesus. She was not looking at the Law. She was looking at Jesus. She did not see him as condemning and hard like the Law. She saw Jesus as a gracious Saviour, overflowing with compassion and mercy. She saw him as the gracious healer and that is who Jesus, the Son of God is. It is how God wants us to see His Son and how He wants us to see Himself. When we do, we will come into the fullness of life Jesus came to give. Jesus commended the woman's faith. He did not condemn her for breaking the Law. God's mercy always triumphs over judgment. It did for the bleeding woman and it does for us today. God does not heal us because we obey the Law. He heals us because we believe that His Son Jesus, who is God died on the cross for our sins and rose again. The kingdom of God is a kingdom of no condemnation. It is the kingdom of healing and forgiveness.

Touch Jesus the healer in faith

The woman who had bled for twelve years knew Jesus could heal and she was determined she was going to get healed by pushing through the crowd and touching the edge of his cloak then she would slip away unnoticed. However, Jesus was not going to allow that to happen. He would not let this woman walk away from him believing that the touch of his clothes had brought about her healing. It is true that when she touched the edge of his cloak she felt healing power in her body as it went out from Jesus into her, but it was not the touch that healed her.

It was the same when the Jews were bitten by snakes in the desert during the Exodus from Egypt to the Promised Land. To be healed from the snake bites, God told them to look at the bronze snake Moses had put on a pole. When they looked they were healed (Numbers 21:4-9). They were obedient. They believed God and took Him at His word and the result was healing. The look made it possible for God to do it. Some put the touch in the place of faith, but the touch did not heal the woman. Her touch demonstrated a living faith, which Jesus commended. Jesus was saying to her (and us), it is not the touch that healed you, but your faith in the touch and your faith in me that healed you.

Many in the crowd touched him that day but did not receive what the bleeding woman received. She was the only one who touched Jesus in faith. It is the same today. Many people throng to him in churches on Sundays. They sing worship songs, say prayers and listen to sermons, but they never touch Jesus in faith. The healing of the bleeding woman shows that all we need to do to receive from Jesus is to reach out and touch him in a definite way, be it for healing; forgiveness; blessing, favour, power to resist temptation or to overcome fear or anxiety in our lives. Reach out and touch him to remove all that stands in the way of personal fulfilment and fullness of life in Christ. Jesus, the Son of God, who is God, has not changed. He still gives himself today as he did when he ministered on Earth. When we touch him in faith, we will receive whatever we desire – Praise God!

It is never too late to come to Jesus

This poor woman had suffered from bleeding for twelve long years. Under the Jewish Law, she had been unclean for all that time. From the time her illness began, she had sought help from many doctors. Over the twelve years, they had taken all her money and left her in a worse condition than when she first came to them. However, we can take encouragement from this woman's experience. There are many sick people today who have suffered from a condition for a very long time. They have tried every doctor and expert there is. However, their condition has not improved. In desperation, they have tried every remedy that is going, but nothing has worked for them. These poor people are in the same position as the woman who had bled for twelve years: life is draining out of them and there is no hope for them.

However, when Jesus Christ, the Son of God came to this Earth, he brought the kingdom of God to mankind. Jesus, the king of the kingdom is 'Christ the Healer.' When he came, he brought hope – hope to all who are sick, diseased, dying, captive, lost, weak, and needing a saviour. This bleeding woman had no hope. She was broke and helpless. She was broke on the inside and broke on the outside – physically and financially. She needed someone who could heal her without cost. Then Jesus came with the Gospel of good news of the kingdom of God. He brought hope. There was hope for this woman (and there is hope for us), where there had never been hope before.

Jesus is the same yesterday, today and forever. He comes to people who are broken, withered, diseased, lame and crippled in all kinds of ways and brings freedom for the captives. He binds up those with broken hearts, minds, spirits and bodies. He opens the eyes of the blind and the ears of the deaf and looses the tongues of the mute. This is Jesus, the Son of God, who is God. He came and died on the cross then rose again. He paid the price for our sin and broke the power of the Curse in our lives. Because of Jesus' sacrifice, sickness, disease, oppression, and death have lost their power in our lives.

Faith comes by hearing

The woman's healing process began when others told her about the healing power of Jesus and his word. Her journey began there and so does ours. She, like us heard about this man, who could be the Christ – God in human form, who preached about the kingdom of God and salvation. When he spoke and ministered to the people they were healed of every sickness and disease. What this woman heard made her believe that if she could get to Jesus, she would be healed.

We come to faith in Jesus in the same way. We hear about him when we go to Church to hear the Gospel and check out to see if Jesus is the Son of God and if he came to Earth in the flesh. We go to see if this hope of eternal life is true. We go to find out if the Son of God died on the cross at Calvary for our sins and for the sins of the world, so that we might have eternal life. We hear first then we go and check it out. Then the more we hear about Jesus, the more faith we have to believe and trust in him not only for our salvation, but also for our healing.

We are healed by believing

It is the same process we follow to be healed by Jesus. We need to hear the word of God, about the healings Jesus performed when he ministered on Earth. We need to hear he still heals today and to listen to testimonies of people who have been healed by him. The more we continue to hear, the more our faith grows to receive our healing from Jesus. Faith comes by hearing and hearing by the word of God.

This woman would have heard Jesus' words and been told that power had come out of him to heal a paralytic in Capernaum (Luke 5:17-26) and when he healed the people before he gave the Sermon on the Mount (Luke 6:17-19). Whatever she saw or heard, it strengthened her faith to such a degree that she believed that if she could get to Jesus and touch the edge of his cloak then she would be healed. Hearing raised her faith and her resolve to get to Jesus and hearing will raise our faith and resolve to get to him as well.

Speak in faith over your sickness

Faith with a purpose says, "I am whole." It does not say, "I don't feel any better." Faith says, "My leg is fine." It does not say, "My leg is lame." Faith does not look at the sickness and say what it sees. It says what it does not see: healing and health. It is the kind of faith that brings about our healing today and it is the kind this woman had. From twelve years of suffering, this woman would have grown weaker. Yet what she heard about Jesus stirred her to the core of her being to push through the crowd to touch him. Many in the crowd touched Jesus that day, but nothing happened to them, because unlike the bleeding woman, they did not touch him in faith. When she touched Jesus in faith, healing power left him and exploded in healing power in her body. If we believe God and push through to touch Him, we will experience His healing power exploding in our bodies and we will be healed at once.

To go to Jesus in the way she did, this woman must have heard how good, kind, loving and able he was and it fired her faith to believe he could and would heal her. She believed Jesus could do what the doctors could not. And the good news for us today is that Jesus has not changed. He is the same now as he was when he healed the bleeding woman. Today, Jesus still does what the doctors cannot do.

The woman was convinced that Jesus had the power to heal her, even though her body showed all the signs of her painful condition. She was able to say in faith, "If only I touch his cloak, I will be healed." She did not experience her healing before she believed, but after – after she put that belief into practise. She believed in Jesus' willingness and ability to heal and she acted in faith. Then she received her healing. In the same way God wants us to believe in His willingness and ability to heal us today. It does not matter how long we have had our illness or how bad it is. He wants us to look at the greater truth of His word and His healing power than the condition of our sickness. Like this woman, when we take our eyes off our ailment and fix them on Jesus – when we reach out to touch him for our healing, we will be healed.

Dignity restored

After Jesus felt the power go out of him to heal her, he asked the crowd who had touched him. When the woman saw that she could not go unnoticed, she fell trembling at his feet and told why she had touched him and how she had been instantly healed. In response Jesus said, *"Daughter, your faith has healed you. Go in peace and be freed from your suffering."* What a beautiful Saviour. He called her, 'daughter'.

He not only restored her health, but also her dignity. He restored her status. In calling her, 'daughter', he was calling her, 'a daughter of Abraham, and of God'. Jesus is so loving and gracious. For twelve years the Law excluded her. *"Daughter,"* was his first word to her. It was instant acceptance. It was restoration at all levels. It is Jesus in all his beauty. It is the beauty of God's kingdom. It is available to all. Come to Jesus! He will heal you and restore your whole life.

The different ways Jesus healed people

Previously, we have seen that Jesus healed the sick with a word or he healed them with a touch or with a word and a touch. There were times when people were healed when the power to heal was present with Jesus, as in the case of the paralytic (Luke 5:17-26). He healed when a centurion came to him in faith, but he came on behalf of his paralysed servant not himself (Matthew 8:5-13). The bleeding woman was the first person to come to Jesus in faith for their own healing.

The Scriptures say that power came out of Jesus to heal her. The healing virtue flowing through him was so great it saturated his clothes. All she had to do was touch his clothes to be healed. She was not conscious of her faith when she touched him, but of Jesus and his grace. When she saw his grace, Jesus saw her faith. When we see his grace we will find faith arises in us to receive what we ask of him. The same healing virtue that flowed through him that day still flows through him today. Reach out in faith and touch him and receive your healing.

Miracle 16

Jesus raised Jairus' daughter

'Whilst he was saying this, a ruler came and knelt before him and said, "My daughter has just died. But come and put your hand on her, and she will live." Jesus went with him, and so did his disciples.

When Jesus entered the ruler's house and saw the flute players and the noisy crowd, he said, "Go away. The girl is not dead, but asleep." But they laughed at him. After the crowd had been put outside, he went in and took the girl by the hand, and she got up. News of this spread through all that region.' – **Matthew 9:18-26**

'When Jesus had again crossed over by boat to the other side of the lake, a large crowd gathered around him while he was by the lake. Then one of the synagogue rulers named Jairus, came there. Seeing Jesus, he fell at his feet and pleaded earnestly with him, "My little daughter is dying. Please come and put your hands on her so that she will be healed and live." So Jesus went with him.

While Jesus was still speaking some men came from the house of Jairus, the synagogue ruler. "Your daughter is dead," they said. "Why bother the teacher anymore?" Ignoring what they said, Jesus told the synagogue ruler, ***"Don't be afraid. Only believe."***

He let no one follow him but Peter, James and his brother John. When he came to Jairus' home, he saw a commotion, with people crying and wailing loudly. He went in and said, "Why all this commotion and wailing? The child is not dead but asleep." But they laughed at him.

After he put them all out, he took the child's father and mother and the disciples who were with him and went in where the child was. He took her by the hand and said to her, "Talitha koum!" (which means, "Little girl, I say to you, get up!"). Immediately the girl stood up and walked around (she was twelve years old). At this they were amazed. He gave strict orders not to let anyone know about this and told them to give her something to eat.' **– Mark 5:21-43**

'Now when Jesus returned, a crowd welcomed him, for they were all expecting him. Then a man named Jairus, a ruler of the synagogue, came and fell at Jesus' feet, pleading with him to come to his house because his only daughter, a girl of about twelve was dying.

While Jesus was still speaking someone came from the house of Jairus, the synagogue ruler. "Your daughter is dead," he said. "Don't bother the teacher anymore."

Hearing this, Jesus said to Jairus, ***"Don't be afraid, only believe, and she will be healed."***

When he arrived at Jairus' house, Jesus did not let anyone go in with him except Peter, John and James and the child's father and mother. Meanwhile, all the people were wailing and mourning for her. "Stop wailing," Jesus said, "She is not dead, but asleep."

They laughed at him, knowing she was dead. But he took her by the hand and said, "My child, get up!" Her spirit returned, and at once she stood up. Then he told them to give her something to eat. Her parents were astonished, but he ordered them not to tell anyone what had happened.' **– Luke 8:40-56**

16. Jesus raised Jairus' daughter

When the bleeding woman touched the edge of Jesus' cloak to be healed, he was on his way to the house of Jairus, the synagogue ruler to heal his dying daughter. He wanted Jesus to put his hands on his daughter to heal her. That was the extent of Jairus' faith. He believed she would be healed only if Jesus laid his hands on her. It contrasts with the faith of the bleeding woman who believed she would be healed if she touched Jesus. When Jairus asked him to come to heal his daughter, he said, "*I will come.*" What a beautiful assurance for Jairus and us. When we ask Jesus for healing, he comes to heal.

Any faith that Jairus might have had was probably shattered right after Jesus had commended the bleeding woman for her faith. As he and Jesus made their way to his home, people came from there to tell him that his daughter had died. But Jesus was not going to let this news affect him. Just like the time he raised the widow's son (Luke 7:11-17), Jesus turned to the one in immediate pain and addressed him. Jesus told Jairus, "*Don't be afraid. Only believe!*"

When it comes to our healing, Jesus' message is the same to us today as it was to Jairus that day, "Don't be afraid. Only believe." He does not want us to be afraid of any sickness, or any disease – not even death, because he knows that in him we have victory over every disease and sickness and even death. That day, Jesus was not going to let any bad news deter him – not even death and we should have the same attitude as well. In fact nothing should deter us if we rely on our identity in Jesus Christ. He wants us to base everything in our lives on our standing in him and not on our circumstances or on anything of ourselves. He wants us to live in the fact that we are loved by God in Christ. We cannot make God love us more by what we do or do not do and we cannot make God love us less by what we do or do not do. And there is nothing that we can say or think or not say or not think that will make Him love us any more or any less. It is God's great love for us.

Don't be afraid. Only believe!

Jesus' ability and willingness to heal are not diminished by anything we do, say or think. If we trust in our standing in Jesus Christ then nothing that happens or is said in this world should deter us from our goal of God's will being done in our lives and bringing glory to His name. This is why Jesus' words to Jairus are his words to us today, *"Don't be afraid. Only believe!"* Jesus Christ, the Son of God is the same today as he was in Jairus' day. When we do our part and believe then Jesus will do his part and heal, even if that means raising the dead to life.

It is vital that we believe and trust the word of God and what Jesus says and not what the world says. The world says one thing, but Jesus says another. The world says it is cancer, disease and death. Jesus speaks healing, deliverance and life. Jesus had the right word for Jairus at the right time. Only he can do that. He is never behind time. When the crisis is at its worst, the pain is at its greatest, the cancer grips the body most tightly then his words come, "Only believe!" When everything seems to have failed and the situation is hopeless, the words of the living God come to us, "Only believe!" And He will give us the faith to believe.

When Jesus arrived at Jairus' house, he found it full of people weeping and mourning. Jesus told them the girl was not dead but asleep. Jesus is the resurrection and the life. He who believes in him lives even if he dies. He who lives and believes in him will never die (John 11:25). Believers may fall asleep, but they do not die. They fall asleep in this world and wake up with Jesus in the next world. They are the words of Jesus, his unchangeable words. It does not matter what we think or what others say, if Jesus said it, it is true and it will come to pass. If we understand this it will change the whole situation. It changes despair to hope as we look to the glorious day when Jesus returns and those who have fallen asleep, God will bring with him. Jesus knew that. It is why he said, *"The girl is not dead, but asleep."* However, he was laughed at by the mourners. How quickly their wailing turned into laughter.

Jesus is Lord of everything

Jesus went into the room where Jairus' daughter was, with Peter, James and John and her father and mother. When he saw her lying there, Jesus told her to get up and she did. At Jesus' word, death had to obey and give back its spoils to the Creator. Jesus looses that which is bound. If we are suffering in our body he will heal us as we pray. Jesus is the same yesterday, today and forever. He says to every sin-sick soul, to every diseased person, "Don't be afraid – Only believe!" He wants us to only believe – to believe only – nothing else. We need to get rid of ourselves and everything else we rely on and have only God behind us then we will reach a place of great reinforcement. If we help ourselves – in the measure we help ourselves – we will find the life of God and the power of God are diminished. Unfortunately, so many of us try to help ourselves. What God wants us to do is to cling to Him, absolutely and entirely. This is God's grand plan for us – only believe. If we believe, we will have absolute rest and total submission.

Conditions on God's side are always beyond our asking or thinking. Conditions on our side cannot reach the other side unless we come to a place where we rest in God's omnipotent plan. Then His plan cannot fail to succeed. Only believe and we will have absolute rest and perfect tranquillity. Then we can say, "God has said it. It cannot fail to be successful." 'All His promises are 'yes' and 'amen' to those who believe' (2 Corinthians 1:20). God's word never fails.

God can work mightily when we persist in believing. We must persist in believing in Him even when discouraged from a human standpoint. We must not be moved by what we see, but only believe and we will have our request. Even when the night is at its darkest, the pain is at its greatest and the disease is manifesting itself at its highest level, we must persist in believing. Then God will bring his healing power into our lives and we will be raised up from our sickbeds and delivered from what is ailing us. Trust in the Lord Jesus Christ and wait on God at all times and in all situations. God will not fail. He cannot fail.

The chosen three

Jesus took only Peter, James and John into the room with him to raise Jairus' daughter to life. He left the other disciples outside. This is one of three occasions during his time of ministry when he took this selected trio of disciples with him into a situation and left the others outside. Jesus did the same thing when he climbed up a mountain and was transfigured before them (Luke 9:28-36). The third time he took Peter, James and John with him was when he prayed in the Garden of Gethsemane on the night before he was crucified (Mark 14:32-42). Two of these three disciples went on to be the leaders in Jesus' Church after his ascension. The other disciple, John based his whole identity on Jesus' love for him and called himself, 'the disciple whom Jesus loved' (John 13:23; John19:26; John 20:2; John 21:7 and John 21:20).

At the healing of Jairus' daughter, Peter, James and John witnessed Jesus was sovereign over death. At the Transfiguration, he showed the three disciples he was superior to death and to the Law, who was represented on that mountain by Moses, and to the Prophets, who was represented on the mountain by Elijah, as they had passed from this life. In the Garden of Gethsemane, the trio witnessed that Jesus was subject to death, and to the anguish and pain of the prospect of death. However, Jesus submitted himself fully to his Father's will and went to the cross – spirit, soul and body in order to fully redeem us – spirit, soul and body. The cross is the centre of God's plan of salvation for mankind, spirit, soul and body. We must look to Jesus. We must look to the cross. We must see the Son of God, who is God dying on the cross for our sins. We must see his wounds. We must see that by his wounds we are healed. If we believe only, we will have our healing from every sickness and every disease and from all that oppresses us.

Miracle 17

Jesus healed two blind men

'As Jesus went on from there, two blind men followed him, calling out, "Have mercy on us, Son of David!"

When he had gone indoors, the blind men came to him, and he asked them, "Do you believe I am able to do this?"

"Yes, Lord," they replied.

Then he touched their eyes and said, "According to your faith will it be done to you" and their sight was restored. Jesus warned them sternly, "See that no one knows about this." But they went out and spread the news about him all over that region.' – **Matthew 9:27-31**

17. Jesus healed two blind men

After Jesus had raised Jairus' daughter to life, he left that house and two blind men followed him, calling out, "*Have mercy on us, Son of David.*" 'Son of David,' is the Jewish name for God's Christ who would redeem Israel from all its oppressors and who would sit on the throne of King David forever. Jesus is God's Christ. The two blind men called him by his official title, yet no sighted person had seen him that way. Two blind men could see what the sighted could not. However, Jesus did not respond to them immediately. Perhaps he wanted to see how determined they were to be healed. They proved their determination by following him inside his (Peter's) home in Capernaum.

Jesus asked the two blind men if they believed he was able to restore their sight. God's Son, who is God asks us the same question today when we call to him for healing. Jesus wants our answer to be the same as the answer the pair gave that day, "*Yes Lord!*" Like them, we must believe he has the power, authority and ability to heal our sicknesses, no matter how bad they are or how long we have had them. Like them, according to our faith, will it be done to us. Like them, Jesus wants us to believe and confess he can heal us because he is the Christ, God's Son. It was that faith and his touch that healed them.

Like the woman who had bled for twelve years, the two blind men came to Jesus in faith for their healing. However, they were the first during his time of ministry that cried out to him for healing. Yet this was not the first time God responded when his people cried out to him. Throughout Israel's history, they repeatedly cried out to God and He was always merciful to their cry. In the Exodus, they cried out to God when they saw the Egyptian army approaching them. He parted the Red Sea for them to pass through on dry ground then brought the waters back on the Egyptians when they followed them into the sea (Exodus 14:10-28). In the Promised Land, repeatedly they cried out for deliverance from their oppressors. Repeatedly God sent judges to deliver them (Judges 2:9-15; Judges 6:7-14 and Judges 10:10-16).

God hears our cry

On all the occasions when the Israelites, the people the Living God had redeemed as His very own cried out to Him, they were steeped in sin as they bowed down and served other gods. However, each time, God was merciful, gracious and loving to them and He sent judges to deliver them from all of their oppressors. How much more then will He deliver Christians, the children of the Living God, those for whom His beloved Son died and who are in Jesus Christ, when they cry out to Him today for deliverance from their sicknesses or infirmities or diseases or anything else that is oppressing them?

When the two blind men cried out to Jesus, he showed them the same faithfulness, grace, love, compassion and mercy that God had shown to Israel throughout their history when he rescued them from their oppressors. Jesus restored their sight. Their cry to him was enough. There are times when a cry from us about our sickness and disease is enough. As the merciful Son of God, Jesus has the power and the authority to heal – no matter what the sickness or disease is or how long we have had it. Jesus is God in human form. When we come to him, we must believe he is the Christ, the Son of God who has the power and authority to heal us. When we do, we will receive from him what we have asked for. We must come to him believing that he is able to do what we are asking for then it will come to pass. It is because of who Jesus is and what he has done for us that we are healed. It is not because of anything we have done.

When the Jews, and the blind men cried out to God, there were no elaborate prayers or eloquent words used to get His attention. There is a time and a place for such prayers and words – when God's children pray to their heavenly Father, the all-powerful; all-seeing; all-knowing God with humility, reverence and respect. In times of great need and great pain a cry from the heart is enough to get God's attention. It was for the Jews in the time of the Judges and for the two blind men in the time of Jesus, and it is enough for us today.

We are blind

This healing is also a metaphor for us. Like the two men, we are spiritually blind until Jesus opens our eyes. We think we know about eternal life – we think we know about God – we think we know about Jesus - we think we know about the Church and we think we know about faith. However, until we see Jesus of Nazareth is God – until we see God in Jesus, we are blind. Until we see the Son of God dying on the cross of Calvary for our sins we are blind.

When we cry out to him, he will graciously open our eyes then we will see. It is only when we admit we are blind to these truths that Jesus is able to help us. Only then will he open our eyes to see. Only when we admit that we cannot open our eyes ourselves and are dependent on him – only then will his healing touch come into our lives. We cannot see properly unless Jesus opens our eyes. We cannot be healed unless we admit that we cannot heal ourselves and that we are dependent on Jesus to do it. Jesus is faithful and he will do it.

Miracle 18

Jesus healed a mute demoniac

'While they were going out, a man who was demon-possessed and could not talk was brought to Jesus. And when the demon was driven out, the man who had been mute spoke. The crowd was amazed and said, "Nothing like this has ever been seen in Israel."

But the Pharisees said, "It is by the prince of demons that he drives out demons."' **– Matthew 9:32-34**

18. Jesus healed a mute demoniac

Twenty-four hours in the life of Jesus

People brought to Jesus a man who was possessed by a demon that had robbed him of his speech. This is the power of evil forces that operate in this world. Jesus said their leader, the Devil, comes only to steal, kill and destroy, but he had come that they may have life and have it more abundantly (John 10:10). This healing shows the fulfilment of his words. The Devil was destroying this man's life by robbing him of his speech. Praise God, Jesus came to destroy the works of the Devil (1 John 3:8). It is what he did when he cast the evil spirit out of the man. Demons are created beings. The created being had to obey its Creator. When Jesus cast out the demon, it had to go. It is another demonstration of the power and authority of Jesus and his word over all the powers of evil. To be healed today, we must believe and trust the power and authority of Jesus and his word over all evil powers.

This healing was the last of six miracles that happened within one twenty-four hour period, spread over two days. They began on the evening of the first day when Jesus calmed a storm on the Sea of Galilee. It would have been the next morning when they landed in the Gerasenes and Jesus drove a legion of demons out of a man. Then they crossed the lake, where Jesus healed a bleeding woman and raised Jairus' daughter from the dead. After that Jesus healed two blind men then he healed a mute demoniac. These six miracles that all took place in one twenty-four hour period are as follows:

Six miracles in twenty-four hours

1. Jesus calmed a storm on the lake (Mark 4:35-41)
2. Jesus cast a legion of demons from a man (Mark 5:1-20)
3. Jesus healed a bleeding woman (Mark 5:24-34)
4. Jesus raised Jairus' daughter (Mark 5:21-23 and 35-43)
5. Jesus healed two blind men (Matthew 9:27-31)
6. Jesus healed a mute demoniac (Matthew 9:32-34)

Jesus' power is available to us all of the time

It shows how busy Jesus was in demonstrating the kingdom of God to Israel. He was never hurried or flurried but used every moment of the day to show people he was the Christ sent by the living God to redeem Israel and the whole world. What a Christ! And Jesus is the same today as he was when he ministered in Israel. His miraculous and healing powers are the same today as they were then. Today, his healing and miraculous powers are available to us twenty-four hours a day as they were then. They are available to us around the clock.

It is interesting that the first miracle in this series of events was Jesus calming the storm. It would seem the storm was the Devil's attempt to stop him casting out a legion of demons from the man in the Gerasenes and performing the other four miracles. Once again, the Devil's powers and the powers of evil were no match against the power and authority that is in Jesus and in his name. Nothing or no one was going to prevent the Son of God fulfilling his God-given purpose in his life or in the lives of those who needed his healing. It was true for all those he healed that day and it is true for us today. Jesus is God. He is the same today as he was yesterday and will be always. He is as powerful today over the powers of evil as he was in that twenty-four hour period.

The man possessed by a demon, which had robbed him of his speech was brought to Jesus. This tells us we must bring our sick to Jesus for healing. Only Matthew recorded this healing and he focused on the responses to Jesus' actions rather than the healing itself. He added that after Jesus cast the demon out and the man could speak, the crowd was amazed and said that "*Nothing like this has ever been seen in Israel.*" However, the legalistic religious leaders were blind to God standing before them and said it was by the Devil that he had driven it out. Jesus healed a man who was mute and enabled him to speak, and Gospel writer, Matthew used this healing to show that those who could speak, used their God-given voices in different ways. The crowd used theirs to praise Jesus and the leaders used theirs to condemn him.

The choice is ours

This healing presents us with a choice. Like the crowd, we can use our voices to praise God or like the Jewish religious leaders we can use our voices to condemn Him. Jesus is the head of the Church and we are his body. Jesus told his disciples (and us) that the things he did, they would do also. In fact they would do even greater things than he had done (John 14:12). And the disciples performed miracles and healings in the Church after Jesus had ascended into heaven and they had been baptised with the Holy Spirit.

Jesus is the same today as he was yesterday and will be tomorrow. He still heals today and he will still heal tomorrow. Healings and miracles should be as commonplace in our churches today as they were in Jesus' time and in the time of the early Church. Like the crowd who saw this healing of the demon-possessed mute, people in our churches today should be saying, "We have never seen anything like this." And by the will and grace of God, they will.

Miracle 19

Paralytic healed in Jerusalem

'Some time later, Jesus went up to Jerusalem for a feast of the Jews. Now there is in Jerusalem near the Sheep Gate a pool which in Aramaic is called Bethesda and which is surrounded by five covered colonnades. Here a great number of disabled people used to lie – the blind, the lame, and the paralysed. One who was there had been an invalid for thirty-eight years. When Jesus saw him lying there and learned he had been in this condition for a long time, he asked him, **"Will you be made whole?"**

"Sir," the invalid replied, "I have no one to help me into the pool when the water is stirred. While I am trying to get in, someone else goes down ahead of me." Jesus said to him, "Get up! Pick up your mat and walk." <u>At once he was healed</u>; he picked up his mat and walked.

The day on which this took place was a Sabbath and so the Jews said to the man who had been healed, "It is the Sabbath; the law forbids you to carry your mat." But he replied, "The man who made me well said to me, 'Pick up your mat and walk.'" So they asked, "Who is this man who told you to pick it up and walk?" The man who was healed had no idea who it was, for Jesus had slipped away into the crowd that was there.

Later Jesus found him at the temple and said to him, "See you are well again top sinning or something worse may happen to you." The man went away and told the Jews that it was Jesus who had made him well.'
– John 5:1-15

19. Paralytic healed in Jerusalem

The man Jesus healed on the Sabbath had been paralysed for thirty-eight years. Interestingly, in the second year of the Exodus, after God freed the Israelites from slavery in Egypt, Moses sent twelve men to explore the Promised Land. Ten of them came back with a bad report and the people rebelled against God. When they planned to elect a new leader to take them back to Egypt, God was so angry, he vowed none of them would enter the Promised Land, but they would die in the desert. In the fortieth year of the Exodus, Israel entered Canaan. By then, all those who had rebelled against God had died in the desert (Numbers 13:1-14:35). For thirty-eight years God's wrath was against those Israelites – from the second, to the fortieth year of the Exodus.

The thirty-eight years of paralysis of the man he healed is a, 'type' for the time God's hand was against the Israelites in the Exodus. Once the evil had been purged from Israel, they entered the Promised Land. Jesus, the one who led them in the desert was now in Israel in the flesh. He brought his kingdom with him and this healing showed the Israelites God's hand was no longer against them. There is forgiveness and healing in God's kingdom, where mercy triumphs over judgment. In His kingdom, the years of rebellion are remembered no more.

Will you be made whole?

The healing shows it does not matter how long we have had our condition when we come to Jesus. He is both able and willing to heal us. We need to repent and change our thinking. When we have had a condition for a long time we can believe we will have it for life and can resign ourselves to that position in life, but not with Jesus. God's Son came to set us free, no matter how long we have been captive to our condition. Jesus' words to the paralytic are his words to us today – to those who are tried and tested. We may say like the paralytic. "I have missed every opportunity until now." Like that man Jesus will ask us, "Will you be made whole?" And if we are willing, he will do it.

If God will extend his mighty power to free paralytics, what mercy will he extend to the redeemed of God whose souls exist forever? There is healing and forgiveness for every sickness and sin in Jesus' blood and deliverance for every captive. Jesus says, "*Come to me all who are weary and heavy burdened and I will give you rest*" (Matthew 11:28). God never intended his children to live in misery due to some affliction that came from the Devil. When Jesus shed his blood and died on the cross, a perfect atonement was made for sickness and sin. Jesus bore our sins away and we are free from them all. We are justified from all things if we dare believe. Jesus himself took up our infirmities and bore our sicknesses. And if we dare believe – by the wounds Jesus suffered when he died on the cross of Calvary, we are healed (Isaiah 53:5).

If God is willing, in His mercy to touch withered limbs with His mighty power, how much more eager is He to deliver us from the Devil's power? It is more needful to be healed of soul sickness than bodily ailments. God is willing and wants to heal both – to heal us within and without. First He gave His word then His Son. None of His promises will fail us. What He says will happen. It is settled in heaven. On Earth the fact must be made manifest in our bodies that He is the God of eternal power. He will do this for us out of His great love for us and because of Jesus' blood and all his death achieved. There is such power in the blood of Jesus Christ to atone for all our sins; to break every curse in our lives; to heal us of every sickness and disease; and to redeem us from all the powers of evil and death.

We are healed and kept by the power of God

When God brought Israel out of Egypt; '*There was no one feeble among their tribes*' (Psalm 105:37). There was no sickness or disease among the whole nation of Israel. They were all healed by the power of God. They were all kept in perfect health by the power of God. And God, who is the same yesterday, today and tomorrow wants a people like that today – a people with no disease and sickness – a people who are in perfect health – and God has both the power and the willingness to do it for us today. Praise His holy name!

Fix your eyes on Jesus

The paralytic was looking to the pool and not to Jesus for healing. He and everyone else there that day saw the pool as their source of healing. They had eyes for the pool, but not for Jesus. When he asked the paralytic if he would be made whole, he took his eyes off the pool and fixed them on Jesus. With his eyes fixed on Jesus, he told him to do the impossible – to rise up, pick up his mat and walk. Jesus' words are Spirit and they are life (John 6:63). His words of life flowed into the paralytic's body and it became strong. The power of Jesus' words moved through him and brought life and health where they had not been before. What was weak and withered became strong and healthy. Jesus' mighty power flowed through his body. He stood up and walked. The power in Jesus' words enabled him to do the very thing his paralysis was stopping him from doing – getting up and walking. At Jesus' word, the paralysis left this man's body after thirty-eight years.

Stop sinning!

Later Jesus found the man in the temple and told him he was well and to stop sinning or something worse may happen to him. Jesus was not implying he would get a more debilitating disease if he continued to sin. He was pointing to the greatest sin – not believing Jesus was who he said he was and had proved when he healed his paralysis. The consequence of that sin – if he continued in his unbelief was greater than paralysis – it was eternal damnation – a life apart from God. But, because he healed him on a Sabbath, the Jews persecuted him. When he said God was his Father they tried to kill him. Their legalistic hearts blinded them to Jesus' love, grace and compassion that he had shown the paralytic. Their legalism paralysed their spirit and prevented them receiving the life Jesus brings. Jesus told the paralytic to do the impossible, *"Rise up and walk!"* This impotent man did the impossible – he began to rise. As he did, he found God's power moving in him and he stood and walked. Faith is the open door through which the Lord Jesus Christ comes into our lives. God saves through the open door of faith and healing comes the same way. Receive your healing!

Miracle 20

Jesus fed the Five Thousand

'When he heard what had happened, he withdrew by boat privately to a solitary place. Hearing of this, the crowds followed him on foot from the towns. When Jesus landed and saw a large crowd, he had compassion on them and healed their sick.

As evening approached, the disciples came to him and said, "This is a remote place, and it's already getting late. Send the crowds away, so they can go to the villages to buy themselves some food."

He replied, "They do not need to go away. You give them something to eat." "We have here only five loaves of bread and two fish," they said.

"Bring them here to me," he said. He directed the people to sit down on the grass. Taking the five loaves and the two fish and looking up to heaven, he gave thanks and broke the loaves. Then he gave them to the disciples and they gave them to the people. They all ate and were satisfied, and the disciples picked up twelve basketfuls of broken pieces that were left over. The number of those who ate was about five thousand men, besides women and children.' – **Matthew 14:13-21**

'The apostles gathered around him and told him all they had done and taught. Then, because so many people were coming and going they did not have a chance to eat, he said, "Come with me by yourselves to a quiet place and get some rest." So they went away by themselves in a boat to a solitary place. But many who saw them leaving recognised them and ran on foot from all the towns and got there ahead of them.

When Jesus landed and saw a large crowd, he had compassion on them, because they were like sheep without a shepherd. So he began teaching them many things. By this time it was late in the day, so his disciples came and said to him, "This is a remote place and it's already very late. Send the people away so they can go to the surrounding countryside and villages and buy themselves something to eat."

But he answered, "You give them something to eat." They said to him, "That would take eight months of a man's wages! Are we to go and spend that much on bread and give it to them to eat?" "How many loaves do you have?" he asked, "Go and see." When they found out, they said, "Five – and two fish."

Jesus directed them to have all the people sit down in groups on the green grass. So they sat in groups of hundreds and fifties. Taking the five loaves and the two fish and looking up to heaven, he gave thanks and broke the loaves. He gave them to his disciples to set before the people. He also divided the two fish among them all. They all ate and were satisfied and the disciples picked up twelve basketfuls of broken pieces of bread and fish. The number of men who had eaten was five thousand, besides women and children.' **– Mark 6:30-44**

'When the apostles returned, they reported to Jesus what they had done. He took them with him and they withdrew by themselves to a town called Bethsaida, but the crowds learned about it and followed him. He welcomed them and spoke to them about the kingdom of God and he healed those who needed healing.

Late in the afternoon the Twelve came to him and said, "Send the crowd away so the people can go to the surrounding villages and countryside and find food and lodging, because we are in a remote place here." He replied, "You give them something to eat." They replied, "We have only five loaves and two fish, unless we go to buy food for all this crowd." (About five thousand men were there).

But he said to his disciples, "Have them sit down in groups of about fifty each." They did so, and everybody sat down. Taking the five loaves and the two fish and looking up to heaven, he gave thanks and broke them. He gave them to his disciples to set before the people. They all ate and were satisfied, and the disciples picked up twelve basketfuls of broken pieces that were left over.' **– Luke 9:10-17**

'Some time after this, Jesus crossed to the far shore of the Sea of Galilee (that is, the Sea of Tiberius), and a great crowd of people followed him, because they had seen all the miraculous signs he had performed on the sick. Then Jesus went up on a mountainside and sat down with his disciples. The Jewish Passover Feast was near.

When he looked and saw a great crowd approaching he asked Philip, "Where shall we buy bread for these people to eat?" He asked this only to test him, for he already had in mind what he was going to do. Philip answered him, "Eight months wages would not buy enough bread for each one to have a bite!" Another of his disciples, Andrew, Simon Peter's brother spoke up "Here is a boy with five small barley loaves and two small fish, but how far will they go among so many?"

Jesus said, "Have the people sit down." There was plenty of grass in that place and the men sat down, about five thousand of them. Jesus took the loaves, gave thanks and distributed to those who were seated as much as they wanted. He did the same with the fish.

When they had all had enough to eat, he said to his disciples, "Gather the pieces that are left over. Let nothing be wasted." So they gathered them and filled twelve baskets with the pieces of the five barley loaves left over by those who had eaten. After the people saw the miraculous sign Jesus did, they began to say, "Surely this is the Prophet who is to come into the world." Jesus, knowing they intended to make him king by force, withdrew again to a mountain by himself.' **– John 6:1-15**

20. Jesus fed the Five Thousand

The Feeding of the Five Thousand is the only miracle that is recorded in all four Gospels. The Holy Spirit inspired the writers to include the miraculous feeding in their accounts of Jesus' ministry, because it is a wonderful demonstration of life in the kingdom of God. When Jesus landed and saw a crowd of five thousand men plus women and children, he had compassion on them because they were like sheep without a shepherd. He welcomed the crowd and spoke to them about the kingdom of God and he healed those who needed healing. Prior to this miracle Jesus had learned that John the Baptist had been beheaded. Plus, he was taking his tired disciples to a quiet spot to rest after they had preached in the towns of Israel. Yet, when a huge crowd arrived, '*Jesus welcomed them.*' This is our God. He always welcomes people. He is never too tired or too busy to welcome all who come to Him. God welcomes us always, because of Jesus' finished work on the cross. God our heavenly Father is always ready to receive us.

Jesus' abundant compassion

This miracle is a wonderful demonstration of Jesus' compassion. He had compassion for this crowd and he has compassion for all people. That day he had compassion to heal all of the sick in the crowd. He had compassion to teach them about life in the kingdom of God. Then he had compassion to feed the people's hunger. Jesus is the same yesterday and today and forever. He still has the same compassion to meet all our needs. That day, by the lake Jesus met all the needs of the people when he provided for all of them; emotionally, spiritually and physically. Emotionally, when he had compassion on them and welcomed them. Spiritually, when he taught them about the kingdom of God and physically, when he fed them with five loaves of bread and two fish. His healing would have healed them at all levels – physically, emotionally and spiritually. It is how Jesus operated then and it is how he operates now. The Son of God, who is God withheld nothing from them and he will withhold nothing from us.

Jesus wants believers to participate in his work

His disciples brought the dilemma of the crowd's hunger to Jesus. When Jesus told them to feed them, he wanted them to participate in his work. Jesus wants us to bring the situations in our lives to him and participate in their solution. He loves to involve his children in his work, but his disciples missed it that day. If they had believed and trusted him, they could have performed this miracle. But they fixed their eyes on the immediate. They saw only a big crowd and a lack of food. He told them to have the crowd sit down in groups of fifty. Five thousand hungry men standing before the disciples made the task of feeding them, overwhelming. With the people seated, the disciples physically stood over their problem, rather than being confronted with it face to face. Splitting the crowd into small groups made distributing the food manageable. We must never miss the simple logic Jesus uses.

Jesus thanked his Father

Then Jesus took the bread and looked up to heaven. His first look was an upward one, to his Father. He was not looking at the crowd or his disciples and their lack of faith or the loaves or even himself. He looked to his Father. He was not looking at the problem, but the solution, the problem solver. He saw it as an opportunity to glorify God. He was not trusting in the bread and fish to feed the people; he was trusting in God. Like Jesus, we must not fix our eyes on the size of our need or on our lack of resources or on ourselves, but we must fix them on God and the inexhaustible abundance of His resources.

Jesus thanked God for the bread then he gave it to his disciples to give to the people. Then Jesus thanked God for the fish and gave it to his disciples to give to the crowd. They distributed it to the crowd and all of the people ate and were satisfied. Yes, all five thousand of them were satisfied. The key to this miracle is Jesus and his giving thanks to God his Father. He knew what his Father was able to do, what He was willing to do, and what He was going to do – feed the crowd with the five loaves and two fish that he held in his hands.

Jesus did not look at the physical as his disciples did and see the size of the problem and the lack of resources. He looked to God who could turn that which was there – the lack of resources (five loaves and two fish) into that which was not there – abundance (enough to feed five thousand men, plus women and children until they were all satisfied) and that is what happened. Jesus thanked His Father for the bread and fish **before** he gave them to the crowd. He had eyes only for God and His glory. Jesus fixed his eyes on God and thanked Him **before** this miracle occurred and not afterwards. So when the miracle took place, all the glory went to God. This is how life operates in His kingdom.

Gospel writer John believed that Jesus giving thanks to his heavenly Father was the key to this miraculous feeding. John says, that the day after Jesus fed the Five Thousand, some boats from Tiberius landed at the spot where the people had eaten the bread **after Jesus had given thanks** (John 6:23). There was no doubt in John's mind that giving thanks to God was the key to this miracle. Like Jesus, we must learn to thank God before our miracle takes place, no matter how big the need. We must fix our eyes on God, not on the size of our need or on our lack. Like Jesus, all we say and do must be for God's glory and we must believe our heavenly Father hears us when we ask of Him.

Jesus said that when we pray we must believe we have received what we have asked our heavenly Father for and not doubt in our hearts then it will be given to us (Mark 11:23-24). If we know God hears us then we have what we have asked for (1 John 5:15). The word of God says it, which means it is settled. We receive it, that is, it is given to us when we ask for it. It is what happened when he fed the Five Thousand. And he does not ask us to do anything that he did not do himself. Jesus knew that his heavenly Father always heard him. We need to embed ourselves in this truth, in the fact that God, our heavenly Father always hears us. He hears us because of Jesus' finished work on the cross. It is nothing to do with how good we are. When Jesus died for our sins, he removed the dividing barrier (sin) between us and God. Now we can come into God's presence to receive what we ask for.

Kingdom distribution

The Feeding of the Five Thousand shows that in the kingdom of God, our heavenly Father cares and provides for all of His children. He feeds them and the subjects of His kingdom participate in the service. This miracle demonstrates the dynamics of distribution in God's kingdom are different to the dynamics of distribution in this world. In God's kingdom, it is not a case of people forming a queue and it is first come, first served. If Jesus had distributed the five loaves and the two fish in a worldly way, it would have seen those at the front of the queue get something to eat, but those at the back would have gone without food that day. In God's kingdom no one goes without. Everyone gets as much as they need and more. They get as much as they can take and more – abundantly more. There is no lack in God's kingdom and there is no unfair distribution. Everyone gets abundantly more than they need. We do not need to be anxious or ask if there will there be enough for everyone or question if the supply will run out or wonder if we will miss out. There is always more than enough, abundantly more than enough in His kingdom. No one misses out in his kingdom – No one!

Kingdom economics

In this world, demand always exceeds supply. In God's kingdom, supply always exceeds demand. It is economics in his kingdom. Heaven does not do worldly economics. To operate in the economics of God's kingdom; we need to repent and change our mindsets. We must stop operating under worldly economics and operate under the economics of His kingdom, where supply outstrips demand – always!

We must take our eyes off the size of our problems and needs in life and fix them on God and His abundant supply. With five loaves and two fish Jesus fed over five thousand men, plus women and children. Everyone ate and was satisfied and twelve baskets were filled with the leftovers. Five loaves and two fish would not fill even one basket. In Jesus' hands they fed over five thousand men, plus women and children and each person ate and was satisfied.

Kingdom multiplication

This is multiplication in the kingdom of God. We must not despise the days of small beginnings. The greatest miracle of provision in the Gospels began with just five small loaves and two small fish. Yet over five thousand people ate and were satisfied and the disciples filled twelve baskets with the pieces that were leftover. In worldly terms it would be impossible for that quantity of bread and fish to feed such a big crowd to the full and to have that much left over. However, with Jesus all things are possible, nothing is impossible. Whatever we place into his hands is multiplied into exceeding abundance – an abundance that is far above and beyond all that we could ask for or imagine (Ephesians 3:20). This is Jesus God's Son. It is life in God's kingdom.

Kingdom abundance

It is no wonder the Feeding of the Five Thousand is the only miracle that is recorded in all four Gospels. It captures everything about God's kingdom. It reveals His abundant and unconditional compassion and. It shows how God always welcomes all who come to Him. In God's kingdom there is healing for all and a willingness to teach His children so they can grow spiritually and become more like His Son, Jesus.

This miracle captures everything about the oneness of the relationship between Jesus and his Father. It reveals the participatory role his disciples play in his kingdom and in his miracles. Most of all, it shows that in God's kingdom there is an abundance of provision – more than enough to meet everyone's needs. What a God! What a kingdom! No wonder Jesus thanked his Father. There is so much to thank Him for. We should always have an attitude of gratitude to God at all times for all that He is and for all that He does and for all that He abundantly provides to us in all situations and at all times. It is no wonder all four writers recorded this wonderful miracle in their Gospels.

Miracle 21

Jesus walked on water

'<u>Immediately</u> Jesus made the disciples get into the boat and go on ahead of him to the other side, while he dismissed the crowd. After he had dismissed them, he went up on a mountainside by himself to pray. When evening came, he was there alone, but the boat was already a considerable distance from land, buffeted by the waves because the wind was against it.

During the fourth watch of the night, Jesus went out to them walking on the lake. When the disciples saw him walking on the lake they were terrified. "It's a ghost," they said and cried out in fear.

But Jesus <u>immediately</u> said, "Take courage! It is I. Do not be afraid."

'Lord if it's you,' Peter replied, "tell me to come to you on the water."

"Come," he said. Then Peter got down out of the boat, walked on the water and came towards Jesus. But when he saw the wind, he was afraid and beginning to sink, cried out, "Lord, save me!"

<u>Immediately</u> Jesus reached out his hand and caught him. "You of little faith," he said, "why did you doubt?"

And when they climbed into the boat, the wind died down. Then those who were in the boat worshipped him, saying, 'Truly you are the Son of God." **– Matthew 14:22-33**

'*Immediately* Jesus made his disciples get into the boat and go on ahead of him to Bethsaida, while he dismissed the crowd. After leaving them he went up on a mountainside to pray.

When evening came, the boat was in the middle of the lake and he was alone on land. He saw the disciples straining at the oars, for the wind was against them. About the fourth watch of the night, he went out to them, walking on the lake. He was about to pass by them, but when they saw him walking on the lake, they thought he was a ghost. They cried out, because they all saw him and were terrified.

Immediately he spoke to them and said, "Take courage! It is I. Don't be afraid." Then he climbed into their boat and the wind died down. They were totally amazed, for they had not understood about the loaves, their hearts were hardened.' – **Mark 6:45-52**

'When evening came, his disciples went down to the lake, where they got into a boat and set off across the lake for Capernaum. By now it was dark and Jesus had not yet joined them. A strong wind was blowing and the waters grew rough. When they had rowed three or three and a half miles, they saw Jesus approaching the boat, walking on the water and they were terrified. But he said to them, "It is I. Don't be afraid." Then they were willing to let him into the boat, and *immediately* the boat reached the shore where they were heading.'
– John 6:16-21

21. Jesus walked on water

Immediately

In the three Gospel versions of this miracle, the writers use the word immediately four times:

1. *Immediately* Jesus made his disciples get in a boat and go on ahead of him to Bethsaida (Mark 6:45)
2. *Immediately* Jesus spoke to them and said, "Take courage! It is I. Don't be afraid." (Mark 6:50)
3. *Immediately* Jesus reached out his hand and caught him (Matthew 14:31)
4. *Immediately* the boat reached the shore where it was heading (John 6:21)

Immediately Jesus made them get in a boat

This miracle began when the disciples got into a boat to cross the lake as evening came. Evenings begin at sunset. If the annual average time of sunsets in Israel is 18:00 Hours, they would have got in the boat then. The miracle ended during the fourth watch of the night. Nights began at 18:00 Hours and ended at 06:00 Hours and they were divided into four equal watches. The fourth watch ran from 03:00 Hours to 06:00 Hours. So this event happened over a period of between nine to twelve hours, yet it is filled with language suggesting immediacy.

Let's see what the Gospels accounts of this miracle reveal about God's timing and what it means to us today. First is says, immediately after Jesus fed the Five Thousand, he made his disciples get in a boat and cross the lake. He had just performed his greatest miracle and the Gospel records imply it was now in the past and they were to move on to the next thing. There is a message here for us as well. After we do great exploits in or for the Lord, we must not dwell on them, but move on to the next one. However, we must take the experience and the lessons we learned from it into the next thing Jesus has planned for us.

Immediately Jesus spoke to them

When the disciples saw Jesus walking on the water they thought it was a ghost and they were terrified. Immediately he spoke to them and said, *"Take courage! It is I. Don't be afraid."* (Mark 6:50-51). Jesus' response to their fear was immediate. The sound of his voice and words dispelled their fear. It enabled them to take their eyes off their circumstances and perceptions and fix them on Jesus. His very presence and words replaced their fear with awe – what a Saviour!

This is the place that God would have us live – with our eyes fixed on Jesus, listening to his voice, witnessing the awesome and the miraculous and not being filled with fear. He wants us to live this way even in the midst of life's fiercest storms. Jesus is always with us even to the end of time (Matthew 28:20). We need to know that when we cry out, Jesus will respond immediately. His words soothe our fears and strengthen us in our weaknesses in times of trial. If we find ourselves being beaten by the winds of life and battered by its waves, we must turn to Jesus and his words to find his rest.

Immediately Jesus reached out his hand

When Peter saw Jesus walking on the water he asked him to tell him to come to him on the water. Jesus said, *"Come!"* At his word, Peter climbed out of the boat and joined him walking on the Sea of Galilee. Peter continued to participate in the miraculous as long as he kept his eyes on Jesus. However, when Peter looked at the wind – when he looked at his circumstances, he began to sink. As he started to go under the surface, he called out to Jesus to save him. Immediately the Lord reached out his hand and caught him. This miracle reveals that like Jesus was with Peter, he is always with us in times of crises. And it does not matter how bad the situation gets, Jesus will never let the events or circumstances of life drown us. His response to us will be immediate, just like it was for Peter. He will reach out his hand and catch us to stop us going under the waves of the circumstances in our lives. What a wonderful Saviour we have in Jesus.

Immediately the boat reached the shore

Only when the disciples realised it was Jesus, did they let him in the boat and immediately it reached the place where they were heading (John 6:20-21). They had struggled for nine hours to row halfway across the lake. When they let Jesus into their boat, the wind ceased, the waves stilled and immediately they reached the place where they were heading. Jesus showed he is Lord of all matter by feeding the Five Thousand with five loaves and two fish. He confirmed it by walking on water. When the boat covered three miles in an instant – Jesus showed he is Lord of time. He is not governed by the rules of nature or time. We must believe this to see his miraculous powers in our lives.

This miracle shows we must let Jesus into our situation before he can bring us to our desired haven. Often we do not let him into our situation and try to sort it out ourselves in our own strength. We strain at the oars as we battle the wind and the waves of life when we try to deal with our difficulties ourselves. This miracle reveals that God's timing is perfect. Jesus sees us in our struggles. His eyes are fixed on us in love and when his timing is right, he comes to us in times of difficulty and soothes our fears and takes us to our desired haven. We must learn to wait on his perfect timing. When the winds of life are at their strongest, the waves are at their highest, the night is at its darkest and the shore is furthest away, we must fix our eyes on Jesus and his words and wait on him. Then the Lord will come to us in his perfect timing.

As the disciples battled against the wind and the waves on the lake for at least nine hours, Jesus spent that time on a mountain praying to his heavenly Father. From this, we learn that we should spend less time battling life and spend more time with God, praying for the strength to deal with life. From the mountain Jesus saw his disciples in the boat in the middle of the lake straining at the oars, because the wind was against them. Then he went to them walking on the water during the fourth watch of the night. Let's stop and examine the logistics of this miracle recorded in the Gospels to see what they reveal.

The logistics of this miracle

Jesus saw the disciples straining at the oars in the middle of the lake. The Sea of Galilee is seven miles wide. Halfway across the lake is three and a half miles away. He saw them straining at the oars from that distance. The wind was against them. In fact it was so strong it buffeted their boat. If they were heading away from Jesus and the wind was against them then the wind would have been blowing directly into his face. However, from his exposed viewpoint on the top of the mountain the Lord Jesus saw them straining at the oars from three and a half miles away with a strong wind blowing in his face.

Then Jesus went out to his disciples, walking on the water during the fourth watch of the night, which ran from 03:00 Hours to 06:00 Hours. Sailors say that the fourth watch is the darkest part of the night. So from the information found in the Gospels, Jesus saw his disciples straining at the oars from three and a half miles away, with a strong wind blowing in his face, during the darkest part of the night. There is no way this could have been seen with the natural eye. This was supernatural vision and it gives a reassuring message to us. There are times when we are in the middle of the lake of life with a strong wind blowing against us as the waves of events buffet our boat. Darkness surrounds us. No matter how hard we struggle; we make no progress. We cannot see God in our situation. It makes us think He does not see us. It makes us question where He is and even wonder if He cares.

God's timing is perfect

The miracle of walking on water shows God sees us in our struggles and does not stand at a distance. He sees us all the time, watching us with such compassion and love. Only when the timing is right (His timing, not ours), He comes to us and makes the impossible possible. When Jesus got into the boat, it reached the place where they were heading (John 6:21). This is Jesus. This is life in his kingdom. When Jesus steps into our situation, he takes us to our desired haven. God's timing is always perfect and His timing in our lives is always perfect.

In this miracle, Jesus' timing was perfect. He had not taken his eyes off them, but they had taken their eyes off him. He used every situation for God's glory and the good of his disciples. He came to them at the time that would bring most glory to God. We must trust God and His timing for the execution and resolution of events in our lives. His timing is perfect. He comes to us in the middle of our situations at just the right time. It may seem like we have been in the furnace of affliction too long and in our timing He should have pulled us out earlier. But God's timing is never a moment too soon or too late. Like everything He is and does, God's timing is perfect. When we know this, it will help us wait patiently on Him at all times. When we know He is refining us and making our faith like polished gold, we will be able to stay in the heat of the situations and rise above them and like Jesus, put them under our feet. Each situation we experience will make us more like God's Son.

This miracle is a parable

The parabolic message in this miracle is so deep and yet so simple and so true. Firstly the disciples were terrified when they saw Jesus walking on the water and thought he was a ghost. They were terrified by what they perceived they had seen rather than what they had actually seen. Sometimes in life when fears or anxieties arise we need to examine whether they are perceptions or realities that are frightening us. The disciples' real fear that night was the possibility of drowning. They were afraid that the wind and waves would get the better of them. Then Jesus came to them walking on the water – walking on top of the very thing that they were afraid would kill them.

And this is the beauty of God's message to us. No matter what situation we are in. No matter how dark things are. No matter how much they threaten to engulf us and drag us under – God sees. Our heavenly Father sees everything that is going on in our lives. He is not watching, waiting for us to mess up to condemn us. He is waiting for the right time to come to us in our situation that will bring Him the most glory and to give us His peace. When we are in the midst of our storms, we must look to Jesus and his words then his peace will come.

Peter walked on water

As Jesus walked on the Sea of Galilee, the water became solid under his feet. The Creator was walking on his creation. Natural laws and the laws of physics say that is not possible. However, this is Jesus, the Son of God, the king of God's kingdom. He operates under kingdom rules, not worldly rules. In the kingdom of God, the supernatural overcomes the natural. The supernatural God was exercising his supernatural ways in the natural world. When Jesus' disciples saw him walking on the water they were terrified and thought he was a ghost. They were looking at a supernatural event with natural eyes and tried to explain it naturally. Like them, we look at situations in our lives in the natural. To live the life Jesus gained for us, we must have a supernatural mindset; an eternal mindset and it will enable us to rule over natural situations.

We become what we fix our eyes on

When Peter saw Jesus walking on water, he asked to join him. When Jesus said, *"Come,"* Peter got out of the boat and walked on water. But when he took his eyes off Jesus to look at the wind, he began to sink. Yet the wind was blowing just as strongly as it was when he got out of the boat. The only thing that had changed was where Peter had fixed his gaze. As long as Peter kept his eyes fixed on Jesus, he did the impossible and walked on water. When he kept his eyes on Jesus, Peter became like his Lord and he did the impossible.

When we fix our eyes on Jesus then we are transformed into his image (2 Corinthians 3:8) and the impossible happens. We are transformed by beholding, not doing. No amount of self-effort could have helped Peter walk on water. The force of the wind had nothing to do with him walking on water. He did it because of Jesus. He only stayed above the waves when he kept his eyes on Jesus. When he looked at the circumstances, when he looked at the wind and waves – the natural, he became like them, that is natural and he sank. If Peter had kept looking at Jesus, at the supernatural – supernatural consequences would have ensued and he would have continued walking on the water.

He should have kept his eyes on Jesus and not his circumstances. Like Peter, we must not look at our insurmountable circumstances. They may be huge. The doctors may have given up hope: the cancer may have been diagnosed as terminal or the disease as incurable. Our husband or wife may have given up on our marriage or given up on us. Our firm may have said we are no longer employable or the bank said they are foreclosing the loan on our home. They are all situations in life, yet are they more insurmountable than walking on water? Looking at Jesus not our situations sounds impractical, yet it is the most powerful thing we can do. It will cause us to reign over any storms that arise in our lives. If obeying Jesus' words and fixing his eyes on him allowed Peter to walk on water then there is no situation in life we will not overcome if we obey Jesus and keep our eyes fixed on him.

Jesus told his disciples, if they had faith as small as a mustard seed, they could tell a mountain, "*Be uprooted and planted in the sea and it would do it*" (Mark 11:23). He used the smallest thing on Earth to show how much faith is needed to move the biggest, immovable object on Earth. If only a tiny amount of faith is needed to move a mountain; then just a tiny amount of faith can move that cancer or sickness or disease or debt or relationship breakdown or any other circumstance in our lives. There is nothing more difficult in life than walking on water. If Jesus did it and Peter did it when he was obedient to his words and kept his eyes fixed on the Lord, there is no situation in life we cannot put under our feet when we are obedient to Jesus' words and we keep our eyes firmly fixed on him. What a victorious Saviour we have.

The more we look at Jesus, the more we become like him. Is that not incentive enough? Is there anyone more loving or compassionate or beautiful or kind or powerful than Jesus? Why would we not want to be like him? If we keep our eyes on Jesus we will become like him. We will be full of health, life, strength, peace, wisdom and joy. '*As Jesus is, so are we in this world*' (1 John 4:17). Jesus, the Son of God is all this and so much more as he sits at the right hand of his Father in heaven and so are we, his children in this world.

Get out of your boat

There are many messages for us in this miracle. Another one is that our place in life with Jesus is not staying in our little boat when the storms of life howl – it is out on the water, walking with him over the waves. Jesus does not want the circumstances of life to drown us. He loves and cares for us too much to let the circumstances of life drown us. He has given us the power and authority to reign over every circumstance in life and he wants us to reign over them. For this to happen, all we need to do is believe and trust in Jesus. The more we believe and trust in him, the more we will crush under our feet the troubles in our lives. Doubt and unbelief hinder his miraculous power working in our lives. If we fix our eyes on our circumstances they will engulf us. If we fix them on Jesus and on his words then we will rise above our circumstances and walk on solid ground and in victory in him. We will reign in life through Jesus, praise God!

Miracle 22

Demoniac daughter healed in Tyre

'Leaving that place Jesus withdrew to the region of Tyre and Sidon. A Canaanite woman from that vicinity came to him, crying out, "Lord, Son of David, have mercy on me! My daughter is suffering terribly from demon-possession."

Jesus did not answer a word. So his disciples came to him and urged him, "Send her away, for she keeps crying out after us."

He answered, "I was sent only to the lost sheep of Israel."

The woman came and knelt before him. "Lord, help me!" she said.

Jesus told the woman, "It is not right to take the children's bread and toss it to their dogs."

"Yes, Lord," she said, "but even the dogs eat the crumbs that fall from their master's table."

Then Jesus answered the woman, "Woman, you have great faith! Your request is granted." And her daughter was healed from that very hour.'
– Matthew 15:21-28

'He left that place and went to the region of Tyre. He entered a house and did not want anyone to know it; but he could not keep his presence secret. In fact, as soon as she heard about him, a lady whose little daughter was possessed by an evil spirit came and fell at his feet.

The woman was a Greek, born in Syrian Phoenicia. She begged Jesus to drive the demon out of her daughter.

"First let the children eat all they want," he told her, "for it is not right to take the children's bread and toss it to their dogs."

"Yes, Lord," she replied, "but even the dogs under the table eat the children's crumbs."

Then he told her, "For such a reply, you may go; the demon has left your daughter."

She went home and found her child lying on the bed and the demon gone.' **– Mark 7:24-30**

22. Demoniac daughter healed in Tyre

A Syro-Phoenician woman wanted Jesus to heal her demonised daughter. She kept calling, *"Lord, Son of David!"* but he ignored her. It is another example of Jesus' response to a request for healing being unusual. He is the God of all compassion and love. However, Jesus chose to ignore this desperate mother's plea. The name she used; 'Son of David' was the term the Jews used for God's Messiah. Yet, she was not a Jew and was not entitled to call him by that name. In her desperation to get her daughter healed, she pretended to be a Jew. She was not coming to Jesus honestly.

Like this lady there are times when we pretend we are something we are not. We project an image of ourselves onto others – the image that we are nice, kind, considerate and loving. We try to hide from view the less nice side of our personalities. But there is great danger in doing this in life. If we do it to the one we will marry, that person will not fall in love with the real us, but with the image of us that we have projected onto them. The result will be – we will never experience true love. If we open only the nice side of ourselves to God, and not who we truly are – warts and all, we will not experience the fullness of His love, peace, joy, rest, strength, grace, blessing, healing and a thousand other things His love brings. Our heavenly Father wants us to come to Him as we are. He loves us as we are. He sent His only Son to die for us as we are in order to bring us into relationship with Him.

It was the message Jesus was conveying to the Syro-Phoenician woman when he spoke to her. He told her he had been sent only to the lost sheep of Israel. It was the commission God had given him. But he was saying to the woman, I know who you are. I know your identity. I know you are not Jewish. Stop pretending to be someone you are not. Be yourself when you come to me. Be yourself when you ask of me. Then he began a dialogue with her that revealed the true heart of this woman and it revealed that she was a woman of great faith who believed that Jesus was the promised Jewish Messiah.

When this woman asked Jesus to heal her daughter, he told her, "*Let the children be filled first for it is not right to take the children's bread and toss it to their dogs*". This woman had set her heart on getting from Jesus what she was after and said, "*Yes Lord, but even the dogs under the table eat the children's crumbs.*" Jesus was stirred by her level of faith and he told her she could go as the demon had left her daughter. She took Jesus at his word and returned home where she found that the demon was gone and her daughter was well.

Jesus' words reveal healing and deliverance are, 'the children's bread.' It is part of their diet. If it is the children's bread then we, as God's children can press in to claim our healing and deliverance. We have a blood-purchased portion of health in Jesus. Today there is bread and there is life and health for every child of God – through his word. God's word can drive every sickness and disease from our bodies.

Healing is our portion in Christ, who himself is our bread, our life, our health, and our all in all. He always receives us when we come to him. His words are Spirit and life to all who receive him. As we receive Jesus as Lord and Saviour, we are born again. His life comes into us. He can so purify our hearts and minds, it transforms us in spirit, soul and body. We become new creations. Jesus' shed blood so perfectly cleanses us of our sins; God himself, the pure, holy God, in the form of the Spirit comes and lives inside us. It is how effectively his blood cleanses us from sin. We become a vessel in which God comes in and abides.

The secret of great faith

This woman and the Centurion (Matthew 8:5-13) are the only ones Jesus commended for having, 'great faith'. They were not Jews, so they were not under the Law, which brings condemnation. As they were not under condemnation they had great faith to believe and receive from him the healing they came for. They came expecting Jesus to heal their loved ones (faith) and they received what they asked for. This lady was not going away until she got it. It was great faith. If we come to Jesus with great faith, we too will receive what we ask for.

Miracle 23

Jesus healed a deaf mute

'Jesus left the vicinity of Tyre and went through Sidon, down to the Sea of Galilee and into the region of the Decapolis (that is the ten cities). There some people brought to him a man who was deaf and could hardly talk, and they begged him to place his hand on the man.

After he took him away from the crowd, Jesus put his fingers into the man's ears. Then he spat and touched the man's tongue. He looked up to heaven and with a deep sigh said to him, "Ephphatha!" (which means, "Be opened!"). At this, the man's ears were opened, his tongue was loosened and he began to speak plainly.

Jesus commanded them not to tell anyone. But the more he did so, the more they kept talking about it. People were overwhelmed with amazement, "He has done everything well," they said, "He even makes the deaf hear and the mute speak."' **– Mark 7:31-37**

23. Jesus healed a deaf mute

In the Decapolis, men brought to Jesus, a man who was deaf and dumb. There was no other remedy for this man. Jesus was their only hope and their faith extended to the degree that they believed he would be healed if Jesus placed his hand on him. He did not do that. He took the man away from the crowd and put his fingers in his ears. He could have said the word or laid hands on him to heal him, but he did not. Putting his fingers in his ears was invasive. Usually we put our fingers in our ears not to hear, which suggests this healing is also a parable. Putting fingers in a deaf man's ears implies double deafness. Was Jesus showing his audience (his disciples) that they were deaf to his words and the spiritual truths of them?

After putting his fingers in his ears, Jesus spat then touched the man's tongue. His touch was specific to the parts of the man that needed healing. His ears needed opening and his tongue needed loosening. Then Jesus looked up to heaven, gave a deep sigh and said, "*Be opened!*" and the man was able to speak and hear. Jesus said what he wanted to see, not what he saw. He did the same thing at Creation. He spoke and made that which was not (the universe) come to be by the power of his word and he made that which was (darkness) disappear. With this healing; where deafness was, Jesus brought hearing. Where muteness was, he brought speech.

Faith calls that which is not as though it is, and that is what Jesus did here. He did this with many of his healings and miracles. He called that which was not there (healing and health) into existence and called that which was there (sickness and disease) into non-existence. Here he used a specific touch and a word to open the man's ears. He spat and used a specific touch and a word to loosen the man's tongue. There are times when our illnesses need a specific touch from our Lord Jesus Christ. We can be confident that when we ask Jesus our Saviour to touch us and heal us – he is faithful and he will do it.

Miracle 24

Jesus fed the Four Thousand

'Jesus left there and went along the Sea of Galilee. He went up on a mountainside and sat down. Great crowds came to him, bringing the lame, the blind, the crippled, the mute and many others, and laid them at his feet and he healed them. The people were amazed when they saw the mute speaking, the crippled made well, the lame walking and the blind seeing. And they praised the God of Israel.

Jesus called his disciples to him and said, "I have compassion for these people; because they have already been with me for three days and have had nothing to eat. I do not want to send them away hungry or they may collapse on the way."

His disciples replied, "Where could we get enough bread in this remote place to feed such a large crowd?"

"How many loaves of bread do you have?" Jesus asked.

"Seven," they replied, "and a few small fish."

He told the crowd to sit down on the ground. Then he took the seven loaves and the fish, and when he had given thanks, he broke them and gave them to the disciples, and they in turn gave them to the people. They all ate and were satisfied. Afterwards the disciples picked up seven basketfuls of broken pieces that were left over. The number of those who ate was four thousand, besides women and children.'
– **Matthew 15:29-39**

'During those days another large crowd gathered. Since they had nothing to eat, Jesus called his disciples to him and said, "I have compassion for these people; they have already been with me three days and have nothing to eat. If I send them home hungry, they will collapse on the way, as some of them have come a long distance."

His disciples answered, "But where in this remote spot can anyone get enough bread to feed them?"

"How many loaves of bread do you have?" Jesus asked.

"Seven," they replied.

He told the crowd to sit down on the ground. When he had taken the seven loaves and given thanks, he broke them and gave them to his disciples to set before the people, and they did so. They had a few small fish as well; he gave thanks for them also and told the disciples to distribute them. The people ate and were satisfied. Afterward the disciples filled up seven basketfuls of broken pieces that were left over. About four thousand men were present.' – **Mark 8:1-9**

24. Jesus fed the Four Thousand

The Feeding of the Four Thousand is a wonderful demonstration of life in the kingdom of God. Crowds came to Jesus and he healed the lame, the blind, the crippled, the mute and many others. He brought the kingdom of heaven to Earth. In his kingdom there is healing and forgiveness. He showed such love and compassion for the people. Jesus cared deeply about them and their needs. He had provided for them spiritually by speaking his word to them. He had provided healing for all who needed it and he would provide for their physical needs by feeding them. Jesus did not want them to come to harm on the way home, because of their lack of food. This miracle shows, in the kingdom of God, He provides for all our needs.

Kingdom distribution

Jesus asked his disciples what they had to feed the people and they gave him seven loaves and a few fish. Jesus took the bread, looked up to heaven and gave thanks to his Father for it and for what He was about to do with it. Then he took the fish and thanked God for it and for what He would do with it. Then he demonstrated kingdom of heaven style distribution. It was not earthly distribution. It was not first come, first served, so please form a long queue. With just seven loaves and a few fish, those at the front of the queue would have received something to eat, but those at the back would have gone without.

In God's kingdom distribution is fair. Everyone gets as much as they need. Everyone gets as much as they are able to take and more – abundantly more. There is no lack of anything for anyone in God's kingdom. There is no need to be anxious or to question whether there will be enough. There is no need to worry about supply running out or to fear missing out. With Jesus there is always more than enough – abundantly more than enough. No one misses out in the kingdom of God – no one. We need to repent and change our mindset regarding God's kindness. We must fix our minds on God's abundant supply (not our lack), which is far above all we could ask for or imagine.

Kingdom participation

Those who belong to God's kingdom participate in His ministering to the needy. God so loves His children that He delights to involve them in the miraculous. This miracle feeding was executed through his disciples, but it began in the hands of Jesus. He took what was given to him and he multiplied it into exceeding abundance – above and beyond all that was needed. And Jesus is still the same today. He takes what we give him and multiplies it into exceeding abundance, beyond all that we could ask for or even imagine.

Kingdom multiplication

Jesus fed four thousand men besides women and children with just seven loaves of bread and a few fish. What is more, everyone ate and was satisfied. Afterwards the disciples filled seven baskets with the pieces that were leftover. This is kingdom multiplication. Seven loaves and a few fish would not fill one basket. Yet from the loaves and fish, Jesus fed four thousand men, plus women and children. So the number could have been more than ten thousand. However, everyone ate and they were all satisfied and seven baskets were filled with the leftover pieces of bread and fish. Jesus did the impossible.

Giving thanks to God the Father

The key to this miraculous feeding was Jesus giving thanks to his Father. Jesus knew what his Father could do. He knew what He was able to do. He knew what He was willing to do and he knew what He was going to do: feed the vast crowd with a few loaves and a few fish. Jesus looked to the One who could turn that which was there (the lack of food) into that which was not there (an abundance of food) and that is what happened that day by the Sea of Galilee. Jesus thanked his heavenly Father for the bread before he gave it to the Four Thousand. He thanked his heavenly Father for the fish before he gave it to the crowd. He thanked his Father before the miracle took place. He did not thank Him whilst it was taking place or after it had taken place. Faith thanks our heavenly Father before the miracle occurs.

God hears us

Jesus knew God always heard him (John 11:41-42). Because of what Jesus did for us on the cross, our heavenly Father always hears us. Yes, it is incredible that God, the Creator of the universe hears us. He does not hear us because of anything we have done. He hears us because He loves us and because His Son died in our place. Jesus paid the price for our sin. He removed the dividing wall between God and us. Do we deserve to be heard? Of course not! Do we deserve to have access to God? No! But because of Jesus we can. His death on the cross has made it possible. If we know God hears us then we know He has given us what we have asked for. That is why we thank God for hearing us. It is not as the miracle happens or after it happens that we thank God – it is before the miracle happens that we thank Him. Knowing we are heard is a greater blessing than the manifestation of God's miracle. Knowing we are heard is the beauty of our relationship with God. He hears us – end of story and we have what we asked for.

This miracle reveals everything about God's kingdom. It shows His love, compassion, care, healing, teaching and abundant provision of needs. It reveals everything about Jesus' relationship with his Father. It reveals everything about his disciples' participatory role in the kingdom of God and in the execution of His miracles and wonders. It reveals the wonderful truth that the recipients of God's abundant provision did absolutely nothing to deserve or earn His kindness.

Jesus did not qualify anyone in the crowd to receive the miraculous feeding that day. He did not divide the crowd into sinners on one side and the religious on the other side. He did not tell anyone they could not eat because they had sinned. Jesus knew his heavenly Father loves to show His kindness and he was not going to stop anyone receiving God's abundant provision that day. He wanted his Father to be glorified in the eyes of everyone. And his desire is the same today. Jesus wants everyone to receive his heavenly Father's kindness and His abundant provision and bring glory to His holy name.

The more we take, the more we leave

Jesus fed the Five Thousand with five loaves and two fish. After everyone had eaten enough, twelve baskets were filled with the leftovers. Jesus fed the Four Thousand with seven loaves and a few fish. After everyone had eaten enough, seven baskets were filled with the leftovers. When he fed the Five Thousand he began with less food, fed more people and filled more baskets with leftovers. Surely there should have been more leftovers after he fed the Four Thousand. Jesus began with more food and fed less people. The answer is, 'yes' in worldly terms, but, 'no' in kingdom of God terms.

The disciples missed this truth (and so do many today) that God has a superabundant supply, one that will never run out. The more we take from what He has in His hands for us – the more we leave. Yes – the more we leave. God does not just replace what is taken, He replaces it with more. It is how God and His kingdom operates – in abundance. Isn't He lovely? More was taken to feed the Five Thousand from the lesser amount (five loaves and two fish) and there were more leftovers (twelve baskets). Less was taken to feed the Four Thousand from the greater amount (seven loaves and a few fish) and there was less leftovers (seven baskets). Kingdom dynamics meant there was more left over after Jesus fed the Five Thousand than when he fed the Four Thousand. More was taken from the initial amount, which meant that there was more left over after he had fed the people.

In the world, demand always exceeds supply. In heaven, supply always exceeds demand. God has a banquet table and invites us into His presence to take as much as we can. He does not want us to be limited by our own small-mindedness. He is the God of abundantly more. He delights when we ask for more and when we take more. God wants us to ask big and to take big. When we take big from God, we leave even more on His table – a table full of healing, blessing, favour, promises, provision, love, grace and life. It is there for us to take because Jesus' death on the cross of Calvary entitles us to all of God's provision.

Miracle 25

Blind man healed in Bethsaida

'They came to Bethsaida and some people brought a blind man and begged Jesus to touch him. He took the blind man by the hand and led him outside the village. When he had spat on the man's eyes and put his hands on him, Jesus asked, "Do you see anything?"

The man who had been blind, looked up and said, "I see people; they look like trees walking around."

Once more Jesus put his hands on the man's eyes. Then his eyes were opened, his sight was restored, and he saw everything clearly. Then he sent him home, saying, "Don't go into the village."' – **Mark 8:22-26**

25. Blind man healed in Bethsaida

Those who brought the blind man believed he could be healed by Jesus' touch, but he took him by the hand and led him out of the village. This is the kingdom of God. This is Jesus Christ our Lord, the king of the kingdom. In his kingdom, he takes the blind by the hand and leads them (Isaiah 42:6-16). Jesus is the Good Shepherd who leads his sheep on level paths to the place of fullness of health and life. He led the blind man away from his familiar surroundings and gave him his undivided attention. There are times when Jesus has to get us away from all that we know in order to minister to us.

To spit in someone's eye

Away from the village, his disciples were the only witnesses to this miracle, which was a parable to them (and to us). Jesus could have healed the blind man with a touch. It was what those who brought the man to Jesus expected and what the man himself expected. However, Jesus chose to spit in the man's eyes. As his disciples were the only other witnesses to this healing, Jesus must have done this to make a point to them. Spitting in someone's eye is a phrase used when the recipient does not appreciate all that the giver is giving.

On the way to Bethsaida, Jesus warned his disciples about the yeast of the Pharisees. They thought he said it because they had brought no bread with them. Having just seen Jesus feed the Four Thousand with seven loaves and a few fish, he asked them, *"Do you still not see or understand? Are your hearts hardened? Do you have eyes, but fail to see, and ears but fail to hear?"* Then he reminded them of the abundance of leftovers after he fed the Five Thousand and the Four Thousand (Mark 8:14-21). So when Jesus spat in the blind man's eyes it was like he was saying to his disciples, "I have shown you all the love, goodness, compassion and abundance of God's kingdom and you still do not understand. After all this time you do not grasp or appreciate what you are seeing and hearing. It is as if you are spitting in my eye."

The message of the second touch

After Jesus spat on the blind man's eyes and put his hands on him, he asked if he could see anything and the man looked up. His first look was an upward one. This is life in the kingdom of God. In it, people are raised up. Jesus takes them by the hand and lifts them up. He lifts up their heads. Their first look is an upward one. Yet after Jesus' first touch, he could not see clearly. To the man, the people looked like trees walking around. Like the disciples, like the Jewish religious leaders and like many of the Jewish people, he could not see clearly that Jesus, God's Messiah was standing right in front of him.

So Jesus put his hands on the man's eyes a second time then he could see clearly. It is the only time Jesus laid hands on someone twice for them to be fully healed. It did not take two attempts to heal him due to Jesus suffering a lack of power or an inability to heal or even that this was a more difficult case of blindness to heal. Jesus did this healing in two stages, to show his disciples that they too were blind. They were blind to the fact that Jesus was the Christ, the Son of God, who was God, and to the fact that the kingdom of God had come.

The disciples had witnessed the dynamics of the kingdom of God on many occasions during Jesus' time of ministry. Those dynamics were best displayed when he fed the Five Thousand and the Four Thousand. At each feeding, he showed the inexhaustible abundance of his Father's provision in the kingdom of heaven – be it through his healing all who were sick in the crowds – or through the words he spoke to the crowds – or the miraculous way he fed the huge crowds with just a few small loaves and a few small fish. Despite witnessing these miracles and participating in them, his disciples failed to see the inexhaustible supply of the kingdom of God, where supply always exceeds demand. They were blind to the truth that the more that is taken from God's table the more that is left behind. These are truths we must not be blind to if we are to receive all that God has for us in Christ Jesus and the abundant supply of His kingdom.

God does not give up on us

Like the blind man, after Jesus spat in his eyes and laid hands on him his disciples could not see clearly who he was. But in the same way that Jesus persisted in his healing of the blind man, he was not going to give up on his disciples. He would persist with them as he had with the blind man, to bring them into the fullness of his life. Jesus could have walked away and left that man with blurred vision, but he was not going to do that and he was not going to walk away from his disciples because they had not seen he was the Son of God.

The parabolic message of this healing was not for the disciples alone. It is a message to us today. We must be sure that when we participate in God's kingdom, we are aware of His abundant provision. When we experience Jesus, we must acknowledge that he is the Son of God, His Messiah, who is God. Also, we must acknowledge God's kindness, goodness, compassion, love, grace, and provision. We must accept God's invitation to His table and take the inexhaustible abundance of all that He offers, in the knowledge that the more that we take, the more that we leave behind. Praise His wonderful name!

The good news is that even if we do not see at first or believe at first that Jesus, the Son of God, who is God, is our crucified and risen Saviour, he will never give up on us. Jesus will persist with us until we reach the fullness of life which he came to give us. Jesus is not the God of the first chance or even the second chance. He is the God of many chances. No matter how many times we miss it – no matter how many times we mess up in life – no matter how many times we fall short, the Son of God will never give up on us. What a truly wonderful Saviour we have in Christ Jesus, our Lord!

Miracle 26

Blind man healed in Jerusalem

'As he went along, he saw a man blind from birth. His disciples asked, "Rabbi, who sinned, this man or his parents, that he was born blind?"

"Neither this man nor his parents sinned," he said, "but this happened so that the work of God might be displayed in his life. As long as it is day, we must do the work of him who sent me. Night is coming, when no one can work. While I am in the world, I am the light of the world."

Having said this, he spat on the ground, made some mud with the saliva, and put it on the man's eyes. "Go," he told him, "wash in the Pool of Siloam" (this word means Sent). So the man went and washed, and came home seeing.

His neighbours and those who had formerly seen him begging asked, "Isn't this the same man who used to sit and beg?" Some claimed that he was and others said, "No, he only looks like him." But he himself insisted, "I am the man."

"How then were your eyes opened?" they demanded.

He said "The man called Jesus made some mud and put it on my eyes. He told me to go to Siloam and wash. I went and washed, then I could see." "Where is this man?" they asked him. "I don't know," he said.

They brought the man who had been blind to the Pharisees. The day Jesus had made the mud and opened the man's eyes was a Sabbath.

Therefore the Pharisees asked him how he had received his sight. "He put mud on my eyes," the man replied, "and I washed, and now I see."

Some of the Pharisees said, "This man is not from God, for he does not keep the Sabbath." But others asked, "How can a sinner do such miraculous signs?" So they were divided.

Finally they turned again to the blind man, "What have you to say about him? It was your eyes he opened."

The man replied, "He is a prophet."

They still did not believe he had been blind and had received his sight until they sent for his parents. "Is this your son?" they asked. "Is this the one you say was born blind? How is it he can now see?"

"We know he is our son," the parents answered, "and we know he was born blind. But how he can see now, or who opened his eyes, we don't know. Ask him. He is of age; he will speak for himself." His parents said this because they were afraid of the Jews, for already the Jews had decided that anyone who acknowledged that Jesus was the Christ would be put out of the synagogue. That was why his parents said, "He is of age; ask him."

A second time they summoned the man who had been blind. "Give glory to God," they said. "We know the man is a sinner."

He replied, "Whether he is a sinner or not, I don't know. One thing I do know. I was blind, but now I see!"

They asked, "What did he do to you? How did he open your eyes?"

He said, "I have told you already and you did not listen. Why do you want to hear it again? Do you want to become his disciples, too?"

Then they hurled insults at him and said, "You are this fellow's disciple! We are disciples of Moses! We know God spoke to Moses, but as for this fellow, we don't even know where he comes from."

The man answered, "Now that is remarkable! You don't know where he comes from, yet he opened my eyes. We know God does not listen to sinners. He listens to the godly man who does his will. Nobody has ever heard of opening the eyes of a man born blind. If this man were not from God, he could do nothing."

To this they replied, "You were steeped in sin at birth; how dare you lecture us!" And they threw him out.

Jesus heard they had thrown him out and when he found him, he asked, "Do you believe in the Son of Man?"

"Who is he, sir?" the man asked. "Tell me, so l that may believe in him."

Jesus said, "You have now seen him; in fact, he is the one speaking with you." Then the man said, "Lord I believe," and he worshipped him.

Jesus said, "For judgment I have come into this world, so that the blind will see and those who see will become blind."

Some Pharisees, who were with him heard him say this and asked, "What? Are we blind too?"

Jesus said, "If you were blind, you would not be guilty of sin, but now you claim you can see; your guilt remains."' – **John 9:1-41**

26. Blind man healed in Jerusalem

As Jesus walked in Jerusalem, he saw a man blind from birth. His disciples asked if he was blind because he or his parents had sinned. Jesus said he had been born blind, so that the works of God might be displayed in his life. His words show this man's blindness was not a result of his sin or sin in his family line. Then Jesus spat on the ground, made some mud with the saliva. He rubbed it into the man's eyes and told him to go and wash in the Pool of Siloam. The man was obedient to Jesus' words. He went and washed then went home seeing.

If the healing of the blind man at Bethsaida was a parable to the disciples then this healing was a parable to the religious leaders. Before it, Jesus declared, "*I am the Light of the World!*" (John 8:1). Next, he healed a man who had lived in darkness all his life. What was true for that blind man physically was true spiritually for the religious leaders of Jesus' day (and for us). Like him, we are born spiritually blind regarding the things of God. We are unable to see the things of God unless Jesus touches us and opens our eyes. And the Jewish religious leaders were in that same condition spiritually.

Repent means to change our minds

Like the leaders, we may be able and intelligent, but this is not a question of intelligence or ability. And like those religious leaders we too were blind. They had no idea of the person of Jesus Christ. They saw him as some uneducated carpenter's son from Galilee. He stood there before them, but they did not see Jesus at all. They had prayed to God for ages for Him to send His Messiah. God answered them and His Christ stood before them, however, they could not see it. Unless God opens our eyes we cannot see Jesus is Lord and God. Things that are obvious to a born-again Christian, the rest of the world cannot see. We were like that. We were not born Christian. We too were born blind. We became a Christian when God, in Jesus Christ opened our eyes. Therefore the first thing we must do when our eyes are opened by God is repent, that is – change our minds.

Until our eyes are opened everything we believed (yes everything) about God was wrong. All we believed about his righteousness and all we believed about ourselves was wrong. The start point of salvation is changing our mind about almost everything. We have to change our mind about: Jesus; God; the Holy Spirit; ourselves; heaven; hell; life after death; righteousness and sin. We are blind to all the truly important things in life. We have to re-think and turn our whole attitude around. We will never be born again until we realise that we were born blind and everything about us has to change.

Our mentality has to change. It is where our salvation begins. It is why Jesus came saying, '*Repent and believe*' (Mark 1:15), The first step in putting our faith in him as our Lord and Saviour is to change our minds. All we learnt by nature, by origin and by where we are coming from in this world is wrong. The answer to life is not in civilisation, education, money, medicine, culture or even religion. It is in the person of Jesus Christ. Unless we see that, unless God opens our eyes, we will never realise the blessing of understanding anything worth understanding. We will be walking in darkness and be putting our trust in all the wrong things. When we realise our blindness, Jesus says if we will listen to him and heed him, he will open our eyes.

Have you been insulted by Jesus?

It is likely Jesus will deal with us in the way he dealt with this blind man. He could have opened his eyes with a word. He did not have to spit on the ground to make mud then rub it in his eyes. Jesus used this healing as a parable to his listeners that day and to us. To get our attention and open our eyes he has to use an offensive way. He has to spit then rub mud in our eyes. It is very insulting. It is like rubbing our faces in the dirt to get us to see. We must let him rub mud in our eyes and insult us, if it means he opens our eyes to him and all he is. It is how he operates. The first thing Jesus does is insults us. He says we are blind and cannot see a thing. The Son of God, who is God is telling us, we do not know what salvation is or understand the things of God. He says we have no idea about forgiveness or being born again.

Jesus is saying we are blind to him, that we cannot see him – we cannot see who he really is. He is insulting us, but he is telling the truth. We cannot see. We are blind. We cannot understand things. He is rubbing mud in our eyes and making us realise how little we see. But this is the way Jesus deals with us. It is the way we are healed of our blindness. We must let Jesus rub mud in our eyes and insult us. We must let him tell us that we are blind and that we know nothing. We must let him tell us that we are spiritually dead and that we do not understand unless he comes and touches us and changes us, otherwise we will never be able to see. The only way to be saved is to let Jesus Christ, the Son of God tell us just how bad our case really is.

Go to the One who is sent

He told the blind man to go and wash in the Pool of Siloam. 'Siloam' means, 'Sent'. He told him to wash and he would see. When we see Jesus is the one sent from God, when we see he is the answer then we wash ourselves in him. We go to the one who was sent. We go to God's Son, the one sent by the Father. When we wash our eyes in Jesus, we start to see and think clearly in the presence of Jesus. He will wash our eyes and we will see he is the Light of the World. We need to abandon our own ideas and all that we were born with. We must re-think and change our minds in every area of our lives. We must go and wash ourselves in Jesus, the Son of God. Then we will see.

Seeing God in Jesus

We must not put our trust in anything or anyone except Jesus as all else is darkness. When we put our trust in him, our eyes are truly opened. Then we begin to see. We see Jesus himself, not just his teachings or miracles. We see Jesus himself is, the Light of the World. He is the one who reveals everything. All revelation, all illumination and all enlightenment are in Jesus. We see that he is not just the son of a carpenter from Galilee. We see God in him. We actually see God in Jesus (John 14:6). We have not seen Jesus until we see God in Jesus. Until we see that Jesus is God and he is the very revelation of the being of God in human form then we are still blind.

The only way we who are natural can relate to the living, invisible God, whom we cannot see or touch is through His Son who took on flesh. God Himself is embodied in His Son. When he rubs dirt in our eyes and we begin to see, we have a different picture of God from the one we had before. If we had a picture of God before, we had no idea what He was like as we had never seen Him in Jesus. We see what God is like by seeing Him in Jesus, in the way he spoke and treated people. We see God in Jesus when he willingly reached out in compassion to touch and heal a leper (Mark 1:40-45). We see God in Jesus when he raised a widow's son and gave him back to his mother (Luke 7:11-17).

When he did not condemn an adulteress (John 8:1-11), we see God in Jesus as he dealt so gently with this woman caught in sin. It is the nature and character of God. Jesus said, "*I am the light of the world.*" God is illuminated in Jesus. We see God perfectly in Jesus. We see that God is so full of love and compassion for everyone, especially the diseased, the grieving, the sick and the disabled. We see God cares deeply for His creation and loves to provide abundantly for them. We see God willingly sent His only beloved Son, Jesus to die in our place for our sins to give us eternal life and fellowship with Him.

Seeing man in Jesus

When Jesus touches us, our eyes are opened and our blindness is taken away, we also see man in Jesus. Jesus is perfectly God and he is perfectly man. Jesus is perfectly human. Sin is not human. It is not the essence of humanity. God did not create the human race to be sinful. If we want to see man as he ought to be, we must see Jesus. The way God wants us to be is the same as Jesus. Look at Jesus the man. There is no sin in him. We do not have to sin to be a man. Look at the man Jesus. He is a man full of God's wisdom and power. When we see Jesus, we see someone who never sinned. We see someone who loved God with all his heart, all his mind, all his soul and all his strength. When we look at Jesus we see man as God created man to be. Jesus is perfect in every way. He is the perfect man and the perfect God and his death perfectly paid for our sins and our healing.

If we want to know what salvation is; if we want our sins forgiven; if we want to know what the purpose of life is; if want to be righteous and put down sin; if we want to know we are going to heaven; if we want power in our lives; if we want to be healed, and to be all we are meant to be and to rise to God's purpose for humanity, we need Jesus. We need the person of Jesus Christ, the Son of God. To know him, we need him to open our eyes, by rubbing mud in them. We need to go and have our eyes washed by the one sent by God to be the Saviour of the World. When we wash ourselves in Jesus, we will see. The first thing we will see is Jesus. We will see he is the everlasting Son of God, who came to save us from our sins. We will understand the cross. We will see Jesus on the cross and God taking all our sin and laying it on him. We will see He punished our sins in him so we do not have to be punished. We will see he bore our sins and sicknesses and rose again without them, so that we do not have to bear our sins and sicknesses.

We will see that if all our sins – past, present and future had not been paid for by Jesus' death and our sicknesses and diseases had not been born away in his body then he would not have been able to rise from the dead. We will see his resurrection confirms he paid the price for all our sins and by his wounds we are healed. Jesus Christ, the Son of God tasted death once and for all, so we do not have to experience it. We will see Jesus ascended to heaven to sit at God's right hand, where he reigns over all sin, sickness and disease and even death. As Jesus is, so are we in this world (1 John 4:17). There is no sickness or disease in Jesus as he reigns at his Father's right hand in heaven, which means sickness and disease cannot remain in our bodies.

We will see things from a spiritual and eternal perspective. As we keep our eyes on Jesus those spiritual truths will manifest in our physical bodies. We will no longer put our trust in politics, money, family, education, health or self. We will put our trust only in Jesus Christ. Then we will have the abundant life he came to bring. It is a life that never ends. It bubbles up inside and fills us to overflowing. We receive his life the moment we believe and it continues forever.

Miracle 27

Jesus raised Lazarus

'*Now a man named Lazarus was sick. He was from Bethany, the village of Mary and her sister Martha. This Mary, whose brother Lazarus now lay sick, was the same one who poured perfume on the Lord and wiped his feet with her hair. So the sisters sent word to Jesus, "Lord, the one you love is sick."*

When he heard this, Jesus said, "This sickness will not end in death. No, it is for God's glory so that God's Son may be glorified through it." Jesus loved Martha, and her sister and Lazarus. Yet when he heard Lazarus was sick, he stayed where he was two more days.

Then he said to his disciples, "Let us go back to Judea," "But Rabbi," they said, "a short while ago the Jews there tried to stone you, and yet you are going back there?" Jesus replied, "Are there not twelve hours of daylight? A man who walks by day will not stumble, for he sees by this world's light. It is when he walks by night that he stumbles, for he has no light." After saying this, he went on to tell them, "Our friend Lazarus has fallen asleep; but I am going there to wake him up."

His disciples replied, "Lord, if he sleeps, then he will get better." Jesus had been speaking of his death, but they thought he meant natural sleep. So he told them plainly, "Lazarus is dead, and for your sake I am glad I was not there, so you may believe. But let us go to him."

Then Thomas (called Didymus) said to the rest of the disciples, "Let us also go, that we may die with him."

On his arrival, Jesus found Lazarus had already been in the tomb for four days. Bethany was less than two miles from Jerusalem and many Jews had come to Martha and Mary to comfort them in the loss of their brother. When Martha heard that Jesus was coming, she went out to meet him, but Mary stayed at home.

"Lord," Martha said to Jesus, "if you had been here, my brother would not have died. However, I know that even now God will give you whatever you ask."

Jesus said to her, "Your brother will rise again." Martha answered, "I know he will rise again in the resurrection at the last day."

Jesus said to her, "I am the resurrection and the life. He who believes in me will live, even though he dies; and whoever lives and believes in me will never die. Do you believe this?"

"Yes, Lord," she told him, "I believe you are the Christ, the Son of God, who was to come into the world."

And after she had said this, she went back and called her sister Mary aside. "The Teacher is here," she said, "and is asking for you." When Mary heard this, she got up quickly and went to him. Jesus had not yet entered the village but was still at the place where Martha had met him. When the Jews who had been with Mary in the house, comforting her, noticed how quickly she got up and went out, they followed her, supposing she was going to the tomb to mourn there.

When Mary reached the place where Jesus was and saw him, she fell at his feet and said, "Lord, if you had been here, my brother would not have died." When Jesus saw her weeping, and the Jews who had come along with her also weeping, he was deeply moved in spirit and troubled and asked, "Where have you laid him?"

"Come and see, Lord," they replied.

Jesus wept. Then the Jews said, "See how he loved him!" But some of them said, "Could not he who opened the eyes of the blind man have kept this man from dying?"

Jesus, once more deeply moved, came to the tomb. It was a cave with a stone laid across the entrance. "Take away the stone," he said. "But, Lord," said Martha, the sister of Lazarus, "by this time there is a bad odour, for he has been there four days."

Jesus replied, "Did I not tell you that if you believed, you would see the glory of God?"

When they had moved the stone away the stone, Jesus looked up and said, "Father, I thank you that you have heard me. I knew that you always hear me, but I said this for the benefit of the people standing here, that they may believe you sent me." When he had said this, he cried out in a loud voice, "Lazarus, come out!" The dead man came out, his hands and feet wrapped with strips of linen and a cloth around his face, Jesus said, "Take off the grave clothes and let him go."

Therefore, many of the Jews who had come to visit Mary and had seen what Jesus did, put their faith in him. But some of them went to the Pharisees and told them what Jesus had done. Then the chief priests and Pharisees called a meeting of the Sanhedrin. "What are we accomplishing?" they asked, "Here is this man performing many miracles. If we let him go on like this, everyone will believe in him and the Romans will come and take away our place and our nation."

Then one of them, named Caiaphas, who was high priest that year, said, "You know nothing! You do not realise it is better for you that one man dies for the people than the whole nation perish." He did not say this on his own, but as high priest that year he prophesied Jesus would die for the Jewish nation, and not only for that nation, but for the scattered children of God, to bring them together and make them one. So from that day they plotted to take his life.' **– John 11:1-53**

27. Jesus raised Lazarus

This account of Jesus raising Lazarus to life is a wonderful insight into his love and its effect. It began with the sisters, Martha and Mary sending word to Jesus that the one he loved was sick (John 11:3). It is clear the sisters knew Jesus loved their brother. When he heard the news he stayed where he was for two more days even though he loved Lazarus and his sisters Martha and Mary (John 11:5-6). It is clear the writer John his disciple knew Jesus loved Lazarus and his sisters. In his Gospel, he calls himself, *'the disciple whom Jesus loved'* five times. (John 13:23; John 19:26; John 20:2; John 21:7 and John 21:20). It is clear John knew he was loved by Jesus and lived in his love. Upon arriving in Bethany, Martha told Jesus, *"Even now God will give you whatever you ask."* (John 11:22). Martha knew God loved Jesus and would give him whatever he asked for. When the Jews saw Jesus weep at the tomb they said, *"See how he loved him."* (John 11:36). So, it was clear to those Jews how much Jesus loved Lazarus.

This account of Jesus raising Lazarus from the dead recorded in John's Gospel is a wonderful testimony of how much Jesus loved the people in his life and how much he was loved. In fact everyone mentioned in this miracle, including the writer who recorded it knew that Jesus loved Lazarus. Jesus is the Son of God who is God. He is the God who loves because God is love. When we see this love of God and encounter His love in Christ Jesus, it melts our hearts, it melts our will and it melts all our stubborn resistance to His purposes for our lives and His purposes being carried out in our lives. It is not the wrath of God or even the fear of His punishment that breaks the stubbornness of our wills and the hardness of our hearts – it is the unconditional and unrelenting love of God, our heavenly Father that breaks our will and softens out hearts. However, that does not occur on only one occasion. God, our heavenly Father floods us with his love continually. It is like waves of the sea rolling onto the shore, softening our hearts again and again to receive His love and give it to others as His will is done in our lives.

More glory for the Father

Though Jesus loved Lazarus and his two sisters, when he heard he was sick, he stayed where he was for two days. His first loyalty was to his Father and to His will. Jesus did not go with Martha and Mary's timing, but with God's timing. If he had gone immediately to Lazarus, this healing may not have been recorded in John's Gospel. Jesus always sought to bring glory to God. Waiting two days brought even greater glory to God. By waiting on God's timing, a greater miracle occurred: a dead man was raised to life and a greater revelation happened: Jesus was revealed as, 'the resurrection and the life'. This miracle helped increase the faith of Martha and the disciples.

Jesus knew those at Lazarus' tomb had not come to the realisation that whatever he asked God would be given to him. Have we come to the realisation that whatever we ask God will be given to us? (Luke 11:9). The moment we pray, heaven is open to us – if it is not open then something is wrong. When it seemed Mary, Martha and all those at the tomb had lost faith, Jesus turned to his Father. He himself knew God heard him always. He said he said this because of those around the tomb. (John 11:41-42). Because he knew his Father heard him always, he knew the dead would come forth. In the face of such supreme faith that counted on God – that counted on the anointing Jesus had received from his Father – death had to give up Lazarus.

We must believe whatever we ask God for, we have received and it will be given to us. We have the same anointing Jesus had: *'You have an unction from the Holy One'* (1 John 2:20). It is an anointing from above. Believe God and it will happen. Speak the word and the bound shall be set free and the sick shall be healed. This anointing came when we were born again. It abides. It is with us (1 John 2:27). It is the same anointing Jesus had: *'God anointed him with the Holy Ghost and power and he went around doing good'* (Acts 10:38). We must have faith for the manifestation of that same anointing.

At times it seems there is a brick wall in front of us and everything is as black as midnight and there is nothing left but confidence in God. What we must do is believe God will not fail – cannot fail. We will get nowhere depending on our feelings. There is something a thousand times better. It is; the pure word of God. If we realise the largeness of His measure, a measure that cannot be exhausted then we will come to know that it pleases Him when we ask for more – much more! It is the much more that our heavenly Father wants us, his children to have – Praise God! He has a plan of healing and it is on the line of perfect confidence in Him and His word. That confidence comes from and through our fellowship with God. We must take time to commune with Jesus. There is a communion with him that is life. It is a life that is better than anything else. We need to get our eyes off our conditions and off our symptoms, no matter how bad they are and get them fixed on Jesus. Then we can pray the prayer of faith and we will receive what we ask for.

"I thank you Father that you have heard me"

If Jesus said, "*I thank you Father that you have heard me,*" whilst Lazarus was still dead then we should be able to say, "I thank you Father that you have heard me," whilst we are still sick. If our Father hears us then we know that He has given us what we have asked for (1 John 5:15). "*You shall have them,*" says Jesus. "You shall have them" is our answer from him and our proof that we have been heard.

In faith, we let the word of God be the voice of God. God did not say our healing begins only after we believe He has heard our prayer. He says, if we ask anything according to His will, He hears us. If this is true, we must believe our prayer has been heard when we pray. Then we can say, "We know we have the request we have asked Him, not because we see the answer, but because God is faithful and He will do it." It is never proper to base our faith on our improvement after prayer, "I am so much better since I was prayed for, I know I will get well." In place of God's promise we have put some other reason for expecting to get well. There is no better reason to believe that we will get well than the word of the living, eternal God.

The improvement in a condition is nowhere near as good a reason for a person to know he will entirely recover as is the promise of God, even though after prayer the person may become fifty percent worse. It honours God to believe Him even when every sense and circumstance contradicts Him. And He promises to honour those who honour Him. Our heavenly Father has promised to respond only to the faith that is produced by and rests in His word or promise.

Some expect to believe they have been heard as soon as they feel better. God did not say He sent better feelings to produce faith then healed them. Psalm 107:2 says, '*He sent His word and healed them*'. God Himself sent His word. We do not have to 'worm' it out of Him. How absurd then it is to doubt His word. Is it not more rational to expect God to keep His promise than to expect Him to break it? Nothing could be more absurd than to allow symptoms or feelings to cause us to doubt the fulfilment of God's promises. To learn how to believe God hears us when we pray is a greater blessing than the healing itself. Then the prayer of faith can be repeated many times for ourselves and others, and our lives can be filled with the fulfilment of God's promises.

"I am the resurrection and the life!"

Martha believed Jesus could have stopped her brother dying. She believed his relationship with God was so good, He would give him whatever he asked. Jesus responded by saying Lazarus would rise again. Martha believed he was referring to the Resurrection that would happen on Judgment Day. Then Jesus declared, "*I am the resurrection and the life*" (John 11:25). He is not the resurrection of the future. He is the resurrection of the here and now. He is the resurrection of today.

Lazarus did not have to wait to be raised. He was coming back to life that day and that was what happened. Jesus' words to Martha are his words to us today. The Son of God is the same, yesterday, today and tomorrow. Jesus is, 'the resurrection and the life' today. He is our resurrection and our life today. Our healing and deliverance from our sickness, disease, oppression and even death is today.

"Roll away the stone!"

Interestingly after Lazarus had been resurrected and life had flown back into him, he remained trapped behind the stone that had been rolled in front of the grave until Jesus said, *"Roll away the stone!"* Mary protested that Lazarus had been dead for four days and there would be a bad odour. Her words did not deter Jesus. He persisted because he knew Lazarus was resurrected from the dead. Even though he was alive, the resurrection life could not flow as long as he was behind the stone. It had to be removed for the resurrection life to come forth. Many have resurrection life, but the stone has not been rolled away in their lives. Before the life can flow, the stone has to be rolled away.

The stone is a picture of the Law (the Ten Commandments), which was written on stone. As long as believers remain under Law, the ministry of condemnation and death binds them. We need to remove the Law that binds them. When the stone was rolled away Lazarus came forth. When we roll the stone of the Law away from people's lives, that is when the glory of God is seen and they experience eternal life and all the benefits of life in the kingdom of God.

People think rolling away the Law will give people a licence to sin. But being under Law has not stopped people sinning. The stone – that is the Law is a hindrance to us coming forth into resurrection life. It stops us coming into the fullness of life that Jesus came to give us – the life for which he died on the cross at Calvary. The Law makes us do in order to receive God's love, salvation, healing and anything else His Son's death gives us. Grace lets us rest in Jesus and receive all the benefits of God's kingdom and the fullness of life that he died for.

Miracle 28

Jesus healed a demonised son

'When they came to the crowd, a man approached Jesus and knelt before him, "Lord, have mercy on my son," he said, "He has seizures and is suffering greatly. He often falls into the fire or into the water. I brought him to your disciples, but they could not heal him."

"O unbelieving and perverse generation," Jesus replied, "how long shall I stay with you? How long shall I put up with you? Bring the boy here to me." Jesus rebuked the demon, and it came out of the boy and he was healed from that moment.

Then the disciples came to Jesus in private and asked, "Why couldn't we drive it out?" He replied, "Because you have so little faith. I tell you the truth, if you have faith as small as a mustard seed, you can say to this mountain, 'Move from here to there' and it will move. Nothing will be impossible for you.'" **– Matthew 17:14-21**

'When they came to the other disciples, they saw a large crowd around them and the teachers of the law arguing with them. As soon as the people saw Jesus, they were overwhelmed with awe and ran to greet him. "What are you arguing with them about?" Jesus asked.

A man in the crowd answered, "Teacher, I brought you my son, who is possessed by a spirit that has robbed him of speech. Whenever it seizes him, it throws him to the ground. He foams at the mouth, gnashes his teeth and becomes rigid. I asked your disciples to drive out the spirit, but they could not."

"O unbelieving generation," Jesus replied, "how long shall I stay with you? How long shall I put up with you? Bring the boy to me." So they brought him. When the spirit saw Jesus, it immediately threw the boy into a convulsion. He fell to the ground and rolled around, foaming at the mouth. Jesus asked the boy's father, "How long has he been like this?" "From childhood," he answered. "It has often thrown him into fire or water to kill him. But if you can do anything, take pity on us and help us." "'If you can'?" said Jesus. "Everything is possible for him who believes." Immediately the boy's father exclaimed, "I do believe; help me overcome my unbelief!"

When Jesus saw that a crowd was running to the scene, he rebuked the evil spirit. "You deaf and mute spirit," he said, "I command you, come out of him and never enter him again." The spirit shrieked, convulsed him violently and came out. The boy looked so much like a corpse many said, "He's dead." But Jesus took him by the hand, lifted him to his feet, and he stood up.

After Jesus had gone indoors, his disciples asked him privately, "Why couldn't we drive it out?" He replied, "This kind can come out only by prayer and fasting.'" – **Mark 9:14-29**

'The next day, when they came down from the mountain, a large crowd met him. A man in the crowd called out, "Teacher, I beg you to look at my son, for he is my only child. A spirit seizes him and he suddenly screams, it throws him into convulsions so that he foams at the mouth. It scarcely ever leaves him and is destroying him. I begged your disciples to drive it out, but they could not."

"O unbelieving and perverse generation," he replied, "how long shall I stay with you, how long shall I put up with you? Bring your son here. Even while the boy was coming, the demon threw him to the ground in a convulsion. But Jesus rebuked the evil spirit, healed the boy and gave him back to his father. And they were all amazed at the greatness of God.' – **Luke 9:37-43**

28. Jesus healed a demonised son

The people who saw Jesus after he descended the Mount of Transfiguration were overwhelmed with wonder and ran to greet him (Mark 9:15). That was not how the Israelites reacted when Moses descended Mount Sinai after receiving the Ten Commandments from God. Moses face was radiant, and the people were afraid to come near him (Exodus 34:29-30). This shows the Law overwhelms people with fear and grace overwhelms people with wonder. The Law came on hard tablets of stone. Grace came in the person of Jesus Christ.

Before Jesus came, there was no hope for this man's demonised son. However, when the Son of God came to planet Earth with his kingdom, he brought healing and deliverance and he brought hope. This man put his hope in Jesus and knew that he was approachable. He brought his demonised son to the source of hope to be healed. During Jesus' time of ministry, the father was not the only one who saw Jesus' grace and brought their loved one to him to be healed:

People who were brought to Jesus to be healed

1. A paralytic in Capernaum (Mark 2:1-12)
2. A demon-possessed mute (Matthew 9:32-34)
3. A demon-possessed blind mute (Matthew 12:22-32)
4. A deaf and dumb man (Mark 7:31-37)
5. A blind man in Bethsaida (Mark 8:22-26)

Throughout his ministry here on Earth, people brought their loved ones to Jesus to be healed. From the accounts in the Gospels it is clear to us that we must bring our loved ones, our friends and our neighbours who are sick, diseased or oppressed to Jesus to be healed. He is still the same today as he was when he ministered in Israel. Just as he received and healed all those who were brought to him in those days, Jesus will receive and heal all who are brought to him today. Jesus delights when we bring our sick to him. He delights to bring glory to his Father and he does that when he heals people.

"Help me overcome my unbelief"

The man brought his son to Jesus. When the evil spirit saw him, he threw the boy to the ground in a convulsion. He rolled around and foamed at the mouth – a final display of rebellion by this created being against its Creator. The father said to Jesus, "*If you can do anything have pity on us.*" He doubted his ability and pleaded pity, not faith. So Jesus addressed this issue, "*If you can? Everything is possible for him who believes.*" After hearing his words, the man changed his language, "*I do believe,*" he said, "*help me overcome my unbelief.*" It was a language the Son of God could respond to. It was the language of faith. After listening to Jesus' words this father moved from doubting to believing. This is the power of Jesus' words.

This healing sets a template for us to use when we come to Jesus for healing. If we lack faith, we can ask him to help us overcome our unbelief. If Jesus could help this distraught father overcome his unbelief then he will help us overcome ours. First, we need to hear the good news of the Gospel of Jesus Christ and how his death on the cross paid for our sins and brought us peace with God. We must hear that in his body on the cross, Jesus not only bore away our sins, but he also bore away our sicknesses and diseases and by his wounds we are healed (Isaiah 53:5). Then we need to read the accounts of all of his healings and miracles recorded in the Gospels. As we continue to read and hear the word of God and as we continue to keep His word before us, we will move from doubt to faith and receive our healing.

We will see his power and authority over disease and oppression – the same power and authority he demonstrated when he cast the demon out of the man's possessed son. It shrieked and convulsed him violently and came out, as Jesus demonstrated his divinity and his power and authority over all the powers of evil. The created being not only recognised its Creator when it threw the boy on the ground, but it had to obey its Creator and leave the boy. When it did, it left him lifeless on the floor and many thought he was dead.

Jesus always raises us up

Then Jesus took the boy by the hand and lifted him up. This is Jesus. This is life in the kingdom of God and this is the king demonstrating life in his kingdom. Jesus always raises people up. Life in his kingdom always raises people up. He raises people up from their sickbeds and even death. He raises people up in life. He raises them to the abundant life, which he came to bring. During his time of ministry on Earth, the demonised son was not the only person that Jesus Christ, the Son of God raised up. These were the other people he raised up:

The people Jesus raised up
1. Peter's mother-in-law (Mark 1:29-31)
2. A paralytic (Mark 2:1-12)
3. A centurion's paralysed servant (Luke 7:1-10)
4. A widow's dead son (Luke 7:11-17)
5. Jairus' dead daughter (Mark 5:21-24 and 35-43)
6. A paralytic in Jerusalem (John 5:1-15)
7. Lazarus (John 11:1-44)

Jesus restores families

The healing shows the kingdom of God is a kingdom of restoration. God, in Jesus, always restores what is lost. In his ministry, Jesus restored health and life to all who came to him or were brought to him. He restores family, as he did when he raised Jairus' daughter to life (Mark 5:21-43); and when he raised a widow's son to life and gave him to his mother (Luke 7:11-17). He did the same when he cast a demon out the daughter of the Syro-Phoenician woman (Mark 7:24-30). When he cast the demon from this boy, he gave him back to his father. He restored peace to the boy and his family and restored the family. It is the beauty of Jesus. He heals and restores at all levels. Disease and sickness affects the individuals and all who love them. When he heals, he restores individuals and those around them. He makes individuals whole. Jesus makes families whole and he makes their lives whole.

"Have faith!"

When the disciples asked Jesus why they could not drive the demon out of the boy, Matthew 17:19-20 says he told them that it was because they had so little faith. Then he told them that if they had faith as small as a mustard seed they could tell a mountain to move from here to there and it would do it. Jesus chose the largest structure in creation to make his point. If a mountain could be moved by a tiny amount of faith, then any other situation or problem in life could be overcome. So Jesus' words to his disciples are his words to us today: "Nothing is impossible for you if you have faith." If we have faith we can tell sickness or disease to move into the invisible and health to move into the visible. And we can do this all in the precious name of Jesus Christ. It is all in his name and in his power and in the power of his name and it is all for his glory. We can participate in this great privilege, not because of anything we have done, but because of everything that Jesus did for us when he died on the cross of Calvary and rose again on the third day.

This was the fourth time Jesus rebuked his disciples for their 'little faith.' The first time was when he calmed the storm on the lake and they thought they would drown (Matthew 8:23-27). The next was when Peter walked on water and began to sink after taking his eyes off Jesus (Matthew 14:28-31). The third time was when the disciples did not see the abundance of God's supply after he had fed the Five Thousand and the Four Thousand (Matthew 16:8). Jesus was not condemning his disciples for their little faith. He wanted them (and us) to have big faith that trusted in the abundance and inexhaustible supply of God's kingdom and His willingness to give.

Miracle 29

Miracle coin in a fish's mouth

'*After Jesus and his disciples arrived in Capernaum, the collectors of the two-drachma tax came to Peter and asked, "Doesn't your teacher pay the temple tax?"*

"Yes, he does," he replied.

When Peter came into the house, Jesus was first to speak. "What do you think, Simon?" he asked. "From whom do the kings of the Earth collect duty and taxes – from their own sons or from others?"

"From others," Peter answered.

"Then the sons are exempt," Jesus said to him. "But so that we may not offend them, go to the lake (the Sea of Galilee) *and throw out your line. Take the first fish that you catch; open its mouth and you will find a four-drachma coin. Take it and give it to them for my tax and yours."'*
– Matthew 17:24-27

29. Miracle coin in a fish's mouth

When Jesus and his disciples returned to Capernaum after he had been transfigured, the collectors of the Temple Tax came to Peter and asked him if Jesus paid their tax. Peter did not ask Jesus, but answered on his behalf and said that he did pay the tax. In the house, Jesus told Peter that the king's sons were exempt from paying taxes. However, he did not want to offend these people, so he told Peter to take a fishing line and go to the Sea of Galilee and throw it in. He said that the first fish he caught would have a four-drachma coin in its mouth, which Peter was to use to pay both of their taxes.

Peter had been a fisherman all his life, but he had never caught a fish with a silver coin in its mouth before. However, Jesus did not want him to reason things out, and he does not want us to reason things out either. Carnal reasoning always lands us in a quagmire of unbelief. Jesus wants us, like Peter to simply obey. What Peter was asked to do was not an easy task, but because Jesus said it, he was going to do it. So he cast his line into the lake. There were thousands of fish in the Sea of Galilee that day and many were hungry. However, every fish had to swim aside and leave the bait alone to let the fish with the coin in its mouth, come up and take the bait.

The words of Jesus are the instructions of faith. It is impossible for anything that Jesus says not to take place. All his words are Spirit and they are life (John 6:63). If we only have faith in Jesus Christ, the Son of God, who is God, we will find that every word that God gives is life. We cannot be in close contact with Jesus and receive his word in simple faith without feeling the effect of it in our bodies and in our spirits and our souls. We must receive his word and like Peter, be obedient to it. It will always be to our advantage and it will always glorify God.

Miracle 30

Jesus healed ten lepers

'Now on his way to Jerusalem, Jesus travelled along the border between Samaria and Galilee. As he was going into a village, ten men who had leprosy met him. They stood at a distance and called out in a loud voice, "Jesus, Master, have pity on us!"

When he saw them, he said, "Go, show yourselves to the priests." And as they went, they were cleansed.

One of them, when he saw he was healed, came back, praising God in a loud voice. The man threw himself at Jesus' feet and thanked him – and he was a Samaritan.

Jesus asked, "Were not all ten cleansed? Where are the other nine? Was no one found to return and give praise to God except this foreigner?" Then he said to him, "Rise and go; your faith has made you well." – **Luke 17:11-19**

30. Jesus healed ten lepers

On the way to Jerusalem, Jesus and his disciples travelled along the border between Galilee and Samaria. Ten lepers called out to Jesus, asking him to have pity on them. In response he told them to show themselves to the priests. As they made their way to the priests, they were cleansed of their leprosy. When one of them saw that he had been healed, he returned to thank Jesus. The other nine continued to follow Jesus' instructions and went to the priests.

At the synagogue, they would have offered the gift for their cleansing that Moses had commanded as a testimony to the priests. Then it was the priests' duty to examine those with leprosy to see if they were totally clean. If they were, the priests would declare the lepers clean then offer the appropriate sacrifice for their cleansing.

In Jesus' day, the Jewish religious leaders and other pious Jews prayed daily to thank God that they were not leprous or Gentile (non-Jewish). On this occasion, Jesus sent the lepers that he had healed to the pious Jewish priests. One of those healed was a Gentile and he was the only one who returned to Jesus praising God. One of the outstanding things throughout Jesus' time of ministry on Earth was, people glorified God in him. This healing is another example of this.

The healed leper returned and threw himself at Jesus' feet and thanked him. This is the only occasion recorded in the Gospels when someone who had been healed by Jesus came and thanked him for their healing. On other occasions in his ministry, many of those he healed recognised their healing, but this man recognised his healer and he thanked and glorified Jesus his healer. Though God had sent His Son in human form to minister to the people of Israel, the Jews did not recognise him, but a Samaritan did. When Jesus saw him thanking and praising him, he commended him for his faith. Like this healed leper, we should always thank and glorify God for all that he has done for us in Christ Jesus.

Cleansing by the priests

Jesus, our Great High Priest did not declare the lepers clean, he made them clean. It took just a word to cleanse them. Again, it showed Jesus' divinity and the power and authority of his word over all diseases – even one as grotesque as leprosy. When he sent the lepers to the priests, they would have arrived at the local synagogue, en-masse. The priests would have learned quickly it was Jesus who had healed them. They could not deny the miracles that Jesus was doing – the evidence was standing there right in front of them. It is the first time in Israel's history any male Jew had been healed of leprosy. 2 Kings 5:1-27 says Naaman was healed of leprosy by Elisha, but he was not Jewish, he was Aramean. Also Moses sister, Miriam was healed of leprosy after God had made her leprous (Numbers 12:1-15).

Cleansed and anointed

The healing of the lepers was a clear sign to the Jewish religious leaders and all Israel that God's promised Messiah had come to his people. Jesus reinforced the good news that the Christ had come by sending not one, but nine Jewish lepers to the priests to declare them clean. He was making it absolutely clear by cleansing these lepers, that he, Jesus of Nazareth was their promised Messiah.

To declare a leper clean, the priest would take two birds and kill one. He would dip the live bird in the dead bird's blood and sprinkle it seven times on the leper, then pronounce him clean. If seven is the number of perfection in the Bible, the blood he sprinkled declared the man perfectly clean. Next the priest would take the blood of the guilt offering and put it on the lobe of the right ear of the one being cleansed, on the thumb of his right hand and on the big toe of his right foot. Then he would pour oil into the palm of his left hand. With his right index finger he would put some of the oil on the lobe of the man's right ear, on the thumb of his right hand and on the big toe of his right foot. The leftover oil he would put on the man's head (Leviticus 13:1-14:32).

The blood of animals is a type of Jesus' shed blood on the cross of Calvary to pay the price for the sins of the world. The blood on the man's ear purified his hearing to hear and receive the truth. The blood on his right thumb meant all he put his hand to would be pure. The blood on his right big toe meant everywhere he went his steps were true. The oil poured on the cleansed leper's head symbolised the anointing of the Holy Spirit. Only three types of men in Israel were anointed with oil under the Old Covenant as recorded in the Bible: kings, priests and prophets. In the New Covenant of God's kingdom, these lepers who were the most unclean of people and were Jewish outcasts were cleansed and received the same anointing that kings, priests and prophets in Israel received. What an elevation these lepers received. And God does the same for us in Jesus. When we believe and receive Jesus as our Saviour and Redeemer, we too are cleansed from all our sin and our status is elevated from the lowest of the low to kings, priests and prophets in the kingdom of God.

This was not the only time Jesus had healed people of their leprosy. At the start of his ministry, a man covered with leprosy fell before Jesus and told him that if he was willing he could make him clean. Jesus was willing. He was so full of compassion that he reached out his hand and touched him and said, *"Be Clean!"* And by Jesus' word, the leper was cleansed (Mark 1:40-45). The healing of the ten lepers shows that one word from Jesus is enough to cleanse leprosy – be it one leper or many. It is the power of Jesus and the power of his word. If he can heal ten lepers of this awful, destructive disease by his word then he can heal whatever disease we or our loved ones are suffering from today.

Miracle 31

Jesus healed a crippled woman

'On a Sabbath Jesus was teaching in one of the synagogues and a woman was there who had been crippled by a spirit for eighteen years. She was bent over and could not straighten up at all. When Jesus saw her, he called her forward and said to her, "Woman, you are set free from your infirmity." Then he put his hands on her, and <u>immediately she straightened up and praised God</u>.

Indignant because Jesus had healed on the Sabbath, the synagogue ruler said to the people, "There are six days for work. So come and be healed on those days, not on the Sabbath."

The Lord answered him, "You hypocrites! Does not each of you on the Sabbath untie your ox or donkey from the stall and lead it out to give it water? Then should not this woman, a daughter of Abraham, whom Satan has kept bound for eighteen long years, be set free on the Sabbath day from what bound her?"

When he said this, all his opponents were humiliated, but the people were delighted with all the wonderful things that Jesus was doing.'
– Luke 13:10-17

31. Jesus healed a crippled woman

Jesus saw this crippled woman in the synagogue and called her forward. Jesus, who loves righteousness and hates wickedness could not walk past this woman in her fallen state and leave her in that state. We have to ask ourselves how many times do we walk past sin or evil and do nothing about it? We are called to follow Jesus and to do the things he did. Jesus came to set the captives free and he set this crippled woman free with a word. When he put his hands on her she immediately straightened up and praised God. Once again, Jesus' actions brought praise and glory to God.

Grace and Law

Because Jesus healed this woman on a Sabbath the synagogue ruler told the people there were six days to do work so they should come to be healed on those days, not on the Sabbath. He and the other Jewish religious leaders believed that healing was work. The Law said work was unlawful on the Sabbath, which meant healing was unlawful (Leviticus 23:3). This synagogue ruler and the other religious leaders were more bound by obeying the Law than this woman was bound by Satan. The Law had the leaders bound. Yet grace, in the person of Jesus Christ set this woman free after eighteen years of captivity.

One of the strong messages of the events Luke recorded in his Gospel is grace triumphs over the Law. Jesus responded to the leader's comments by saying that each Sabbath, men untied their donkey or ox from its stall and led it out to be fed and watered. If they could do that for their animal, why should this woman not be freed from what had bound her? Interestingly Jesus said that it was Satan who had bound her for eighteen years. It does not matter what he has bound – Jesus is able to loose. It does not matter what Satan has loosed; Jesus is able to bind it. In Jesus, we have authority and power to loose what Satan has bound and to bind what he has loosed. It is not because of anything that we have done. It is because of what Jesus did for us when he died on the cross and rose again on the third day.

Standing restored

It does not matter if someone has been bound for twelve years, like the bleeding woman (Mark 5:21-34) or for eighteen years like this crippled woman or for thirty-eight years like the paralysed man in Jerusalem (John 5:1-15), he was able to loose them all. What an encouragement this is for those of us today who have been bound by a sickness or disease for many years. Jesus is able and will heal us.

When Jesus healed this lady, he showed his divinity and his power and authority over the Devil. Also he showed his great compassion and love. This woman had been crippled for eighteen years. Her condition may have caused her to wonder if God really cared about her or His people. Then Jesus came into her life. First, he called her, 'daughter of Abraham' then he set her free! He declared publicly her Jewish lineage to Abraham. This is the beauty of Jesus. He not only heals and restores physically, but he also heals and restores at all levels. No wonder this woman praised God after Jesus restored her status as well as her health. Indeed, He is most worthy of praise.

This is Jesus and his kingdom, where the humble are exalted and the exalted are humbled. What an insight into the heart of Jesus. It encourages us to come to him and ask, "Why shouldn't we be loosed from what has bound us for so long?" This is the heart of God. He wants us to be loosed from what binds us. If we want to be loosed then we want what He wants and are asking according to His will. If we ask for anything according to His will then we have already received what we have asked for (1 John 5:14). So after eighteen years of staring at the ground, the first thing this woman saw when Jesus raised her up was his beautiful face. This is Jesus. He always lifts us up. The only way with Jesus is up. The only way for the flesh is down. The king of God's kingdom always lifts up our heads. Jesus is, 'the lifter up of our heads.' It is what he does. It does not matter how long we have been bound, He is willing and he is able to set us free. And when Jesus, the Son of God sets us free, we are free indeed (John 8:36).

Complete restoration

What a beautiful sight to behold when this woman could finally raise her head after eighteen years of staring at people's feet. The first thing she saw was the radiant, pure, holy, beautiful, kind, loving face of Jesus. She saw the face of God, because anyone who has seen Jesus has seen God (John 14:9). When Jesus lifts up our heads, we too see his divinity, his beauty and his love for us. He lifted up her head as he restored her physically. He called her, 'daughter of Abraham' as he restored her status. Then he healed her emotionally as he restored her to the family of God. Jesus restored her at every level, through his love, grace, power and compassion. He does the same for us. When he lifts up our heads and we see his divinity, his beauty and his love for us; his healing flows into us. Jesus' healing is so much more than physical. It is full, complete and life-changing at every level.

When we look at Jesus in this healing and see the compassion and love he had for this crippled woman, we see that it was not and is not for her alone, but for all of us. He has the same level of love for every person on Earth. He is as willing to heal every sick person today as he was to heal the crippled woman that day in the synagogue. He is the same today as he was then. This woman did nothing to qualify for his healing and we need no qualification to be healed by him. It was all through his love and his grace. In fact her only qualification was to be in need of healing and it is the only qualification we need as well.

Come to Jesus and freely receive all he has to give you. His desire to give to us is so much greater than our desire to ask of him. Come to Jesus. Ask him and believe he will do it. He is love and he is healing. He is life and he is restoration. He is eternal and he is salvation. He will provide our every need far above all that we could ever ask for or imagine. Jesus Christ is a wonderful Saviour!

Miracle 32

Jesus healed a man with dropsy

'One Sabbath, when Jesus went to eat in the house of a prominent Pharisee, he was being carefully watched. There in front of him was a man suffering from dropsy. Jesus asked the Pharisees and the experts in the law, "Is it lawful to heal on the Sabbath or not?" But they remained silent. So taking hold of the man, he healed him and sent him away.

Then he asked them, "If one of you has a son or an ox that falls into a well on the Sabbath day, will you not immediately pull him out?" And they had nothing to say.' – **Luke 14:1-6**

32. Jesus healed man with dropsy

This healing of the man with dropsy is the last of seven healings that Jesus performed on the Sabbath during his time of ministry that are recorded in the Gospels. The other six are:

Healings Jesus performed on a Sabbath

1. Demoniac healed in the synagogue (Mark 1:21-28)
2. Jesus healed Peter's mother-in-law (Mark 1:29-31)
3. A man's hand healed in the synagogue (Mark 3:1-6)
4. Jesus healed a paralytic in Jerusalem (John 5:1-15)
5. Jesus healed a blind man in Jerusalem (John 9:1-41)
6. Jesus healed a cripple in a synagogue (Luke 13:10-17)

God created the universe in six days and on the seventh day he rested (Genesis 2:1-3). God instituted the Sabbath as a day of rest for man (Exodus 20:8-12). Due to their conditions, the Sabbath was not a day of rest for the demoniac in Capernaum; Peter's mother-in-law; the man with a shrivelled hand in the synagogue; the paralytic; and the blind man in Jerusalem; and the crippled woman in the synagogue. Nor was it a day of rest for the man with dropsy. No one whose body is being ravaged by disease or sickness or is incapacitated by an infirmity or by spiritual oppression is at rest. Jesus, the Lord of the Sabbath could not leave anyone in a state of unrest or dis-ease on the Sabbath.

Jesus came in the flesh to die on the cross of Calvary to give us rest. He came to give us his rest, his Sabbath rest. It is rest from all our struggling and striving. It is rest from all the consequences of the Curse and it is rest from ill health, sickness and disease. If it meant he had to bring that rest on the holy day, nothing was going to stop him. Jesus came to set the captives free and that is just what he did. He did it seven days a week. When he healed the paralytic in Jerusalem he told the Jews he and his Father were always at their work – even on the Sabbath. Jesus is healing. It is who he is. He is healing, not just from Sunday to Friday, but seven days a week.

When we rest – God works

The seven events show God heals on the Sabbath. It is man's day of rest. Healing is not man's work; it is God's work. On these seven occasions, when man rested, God worked and healed the sick. It shows us that when we rest God works in our lives. When we try to heal ourselves and strive to live in our own strength or achieve for our own glory or try to earn God's love through our own work and efforts or try to justify ourselves through our own righteousness, God rests. If we want God to work in our lives then we must rest – in Him.

How do we rest in Him? We trust in Jesus' finished work on the cross. We trust what God says about what His Son's death achieved for us. We trust his shed blood is sufficient to cleanse us from all our sins, past present and future. We believe that on the cross, Jesus became our sin and we became his righteousness. We trust that by dying on a tree in our place he freed us from all the curses of a fallen world and by his wounds we are healed. It is how we enter his rest. It is the peace Jesus gives that passes all understanding. It is the rest he promises us when we come to him (Matthew 11:28-30). The good news is, that in Jesus Christ, we have peace with God and rest for our souls. When our souls are at rest with God, we have life to the full.

Opposition to Jesus

Because Jesus healed on Sabbaths, his enemies wanted to use it as a charge against him in order to put him to death. As he dined at this Pharisees' house, he was being carefully watched. It was not a friendly environment. When men operate with a religious and legalistic mindset they become judgmental, accusatory and condemnatory. They wait for people to fail so that they can accuse and condemn them. Their hearts become hard, like the stones the Law was written on. Compassion and love go out of the window. Any willingness to help someone who fails or falls disappears. Any desire to want the best for others vanishes. Only the Law and keeping every part of it was important to these legalistic religious leaders. Only then would their lives be perfect.

However, for them, to keep all of the Law was impossible. Yet they would condemn anyone else who could not keep it. There was only one person who could keep all of the Law and he was seated with them at their table. As the leaders sat around trying to be perfect, Jesus' attention was drawn to the one man who was physically far from perfect. When he addressed these legalistic leaders, he used legal language. He asked them if it was lawful to heal on the Sabbath or not. The Law came through Moses – grace came through the person of Jesus Christ. It is a wonderful picture that Luke conveys in his account of this healing. Here is grace, in person sitting before the eyes of the legalistic leaders. Jesus wanted to demonstrate how grace can be exercised without breaking the Law. The leaders were having none of it and they refused to answer Jesus' question.

Jesus was not going to let them or their legalism stop him fulfilling his God-given purpose of setting captives free. So, out of his heart full of compassion and love, he took hold of the man with dropsy and healed him. How lovely. Jesus was not going to be affected by the Jewish religious leaders' accusatory and condemnatory ways as they carefully watched him. Nothing was going to stop Jesus showing kindness to this man. Jesus took hold of him and in his hands the man's dropsy was healed. He embraced the one who was sick and rebuked the ones that were proud. This is life in the kingdom of God where the humble are lifted up and the proud are humbled.

When Jesus was here on Earth, his arms were open to embrace the diseased, the sick, the demonised and the captives. In his hands, sickness and disease departed – demons fled and freedom came to the captives. Since Jesus is the same yesterday, today and forever then disease and sickness and all forms of evil have to depart and the captives go free. When we come to him, we too will find his arms are open wide to embrace us and his heart is full of love for us and filled with compassion to see us set free from all that oppresses us. What a wonderful Saviour we have in Jesus Christ our Lord.

Miracle 33

Jesus healed two blind men

'As Jesus and his disciples left Jericho, a large crowd followed him. When two blind me sitting by the roadside heard that Jesus was going by, they shouted, "Lord, Son of David, have mercy on us!"

The crowd scolded them and told them to be quiet, but they shouted all the louder, "Lord, Son of David, have mercy on us!"

Jesus stopped and called them. "What do you want me to do for you?" he asked the two blind men.

"Lord," they answered, "we want our sight."

He had compassion on them and touched their eyes. <u>Immediately they received their sight</u> and followed him.' – **Matthew 20:29-34**

'As Jesus and his disciples, together with a large crowd, were leaving Jericho, a blind man, Bartimaeus (the son of Timaeus), was sitting by the roadside begging. When he heard that it was Jesus of Nazareth, he began to shout, "Jesus, Son of David, have mercy on me!"

Many rebuked him and told him to be quiet, but he shouted all the more, "Son of David, have mercy on me!"

Jesus stopped and said, "Call him." So they called the man, "Cheer up! On your feet! He's calling you." Throwing his cloak aside, he jumped to his feet and came to Jesus.

"What do you want me to do for you?" Jesus asked.

The blind man said, "Rabbi, I want to see."

He said, "Go, your faith has healed you." <u>Immediately he received his sight</u> and followed Jesus along the road.' **– Mark 10:46-52**

'As Jesus approached Jericho, a blind man was sitting by the roadside begging. When he heard the crowd going by, he asked what was happening. They said, "Jesus of Nazareth is passing by."

He called out, "Jesus, Son of David, have mercy on me!"

Those who led the way rebuked him and told him to be quiet, but he shouted all the more, "Son of David, have mercy on me!"

Jesus stopped and ordered the man to be brought to him. When he came near, Jesus asked him, "What do you want me to do for you?"

"Lord, I want to see," he replied.

Jesus said to him, "Receive your sight; your faith has healed you." <u>Immediately he received his sight</u> and followed him, praising God. When the people saw it, they also praised God.' **– Luke 18:35-43**

33. Jesus healed two blind men

On Jesus' final journey to Jerusalem and the cross of Calvary, he and his disciples visited Jericho. As they left the city, he passed two blind beggars, one of whom was named Bartimaeus. They shouted, "*Jesus, Son of David, have mercy on us!*" The crowd travelling with Jesus rebuked them, but they shouted louder, "*Lord, Son of David, have mercy on us!*" 'Son of David,' is the Jewish name for God's Christ, the one He would send to save His people.

That day, two blind men saw Jesus was the promised Messiah – who came from King David's family line and would reign forever over Israel (2 Samuel 7:12-17). However, those who could see Jesus as he walked with them were blind to his true identity. Seeing Jesus of Nazareth is the Son of God and that he is God is not something we see by natural sight. It takes revelation from God Himself in our innermost being to see and to know that Jesus is God. Bartimaeus and the other man saw this whilst they were blind. They saw that Jesus was Lord in their hearts before they saw him physically with their eyes.

God stood still

When Jesus heard Bartimaeus call, he stood still. A blind beggar's cry made the God of creation, who flung the stars into space, stand still. It was not a rich or perfect man who made him stand still, but a blind beggar. If Jesus stopped for him, we will certainly get his attention when we cry out to him. What an accessible and loving God we have. Today, Jesus still has the same heart to seek and save the lost and set the captives free as he did then. Like us, blind Bartimaeus could not see Jesus physically, but like him we can see and know in our innermost being that he is God's Son who became a man and died on a cross for our sins. We know he was buried and rose on the third day and ascended to heaven where he sits at God's right hand in our innermost being, yet we have never seen any of it visibly. It comes by revelation from God. It is nothing in ourselves that achieves this.

Casting aside our cloaks

When the people in the crowd told blind Bartimaeus that Jesus was calling him, he threw aside his cloak, jumped to his feet and came to him. What an immediate response to Jesus' call. He threw aside all that he had and hurried to Jesus. In Bible times a man's cloak was his security. For the poor (and Bartimaeus the blind beggar was poor – Mark 10:46), it was the only thing they had to keep them warm at night. That is why God told the Jews that when they took a man's cloak as security they had to return it to him at the end of the day in order for him to stay warm at night (Exodus 22:26).

So after calling out to Jesus and getting a response, Bartimaeus threw aside his security. He cast aside all he had and all he was holding onto to come to Jesus open-handed to receive all the Lord had to give him. By this action it is clear that blind Bartimaeus was not going to go back from Jesus the same way he had come to him. God desires the same action from us. Our heavenly Father wants us to cast aside all our security. He wants us to let go of everything that we are holding onto in this world and come to his beloved Son, Jesus Christ. God wants us to let go of everything that we are relying on in this world, in others and in ourselves and come to Him. What wonderful love and acceptance.

When we come to Him empty-handed then we can receive Jesus and we can receive all that he died on the cross of Calvary to give us. We need to throw aside our self-sufficiency and run to him with open hands, open hearts and open lives. When we do, Jesus will fill our hearts, fill our hands and fill our lives to overflowing. When we respond to the call of God in our lives and enter into the kingdom of God – when we surrender our lives and all that is in them to Jesus and the kingdom of God – then we will receive all the fullness of kingdom life. This is the abundant life that Jesus came to this Earth in the form of a man to bring to men and women. When God in Jesus calls us to this life and our eyes are opened then we too will never return to where we came from.

What do you want me to do for you?

When Bartimaeus approached Jesus, the Lord asked him, *"What do you want me to do for you?"* This is the living God, in human form, asking a blind beggar, one of the lowest members of society (in the world's eyes, not in God's eyes): *"What will you have me do for you?"* What wonderful humility and loving kindness, Jesus showed that day. Even though he was blind, Bartimaeus saw that Jesus was the one sent by God. He saw that Jesus had come to serve. He asked Jesus to serve him the children's bread. He was asking, "Will you serve me healing – for that is your bread – it is the bread with which you, the Christ feed the children of Israel?" (Mark 7:25-30). In response, Jesus told Bartimaeus to go as his faith had healed him and immediately this blind man received his sight and followed Jesus.

When Bartimaeus told Jesus he wanted to receive his sight, he believed that Jesus was able to do what he asked of him. Then he received his sight according to his faith. When we come to Jesus we must be prepared to answer the question, "What do you want me to do for you?" There are times when we come to Jesus that we must be very clear about what we want him to do for us. But, before we ask him for anything, we must be certain that he is who he says he is and that he is able and willing to do what we ask of him. When we are assured of this truth, like Bartimaeus it will be done for us 'according to our faith'.

Like Bartimaeus, it does not matter where we are coming from when we come to Jesus and ask him for healing, or anything else that we need in life. Like blind Bartimaeus, there is nothing in our background, our ancestry or our circumstances that disqualify us from coming to Jesus Christ, the Son of God, who is God and receiving what we ask him to give us. What Grace! What a loving, humble Saviour we serve – one who is willing to stop in his tracks when we call him – one who is willing to embrace us in our fallen, sick and diseased state – one who is willing to heal us when we call out to him and come to him for healing.

Follow Jesus!

As soon as Bartimaeus' sight was restored he followed Jesus. He did not need teaching about the kingdom of God to follow Jesus – he had experienced life in the kingdom first hand. Once again it was the kindness of God in this healing that led this man to repent. Bartimaeus changed his mind when he experienced the kindness of God in Christ Jesus to heal him of his blindness. When he saw the humility of God in human form who stopped when this blind beggar called him, it not only caused him to repent and change his mind, but it also changed his heart and it changed his life as he followed Jesus his healer. He followed the Son of David. He followed the one he believed was the Christ, who would sit on the throne of David and reign for all eternity. We like Bartimaeus should follow Jesus in the same way when we experience the kindness of God in his Son, Jesus, our Saviour.

Miracle 34

Jesus cursed a fig tree

'Early in the morning, on his way back to the city, Jesus was hungry. Seeing a fig tree by the road, he went up to it, but found nothing on it except leaves. He said to it, "May you never bear fruit again!" <u>Immediately the tree withered</u>. When the disciples saw this, they were amazed. "How did the fig tree wither so quickly?" they asked. He said, "I tell you the truth, if you have faith and do not doubt; not only can you do what was done to the fig tree, but also you can say to this mountain, "Go, throw yourself into the sea," and it will be done. If you believe, you will receive whatever you ask for in prayer."' – **Matthew 21:18-22**

'The next day as they were leaving Bethany, Jesus was hungry. Seeing in the distance a fig tree in leaf, he went to find out if it had any fruit. When he reached it, he found nothing but leaves because it was not the season for figs. Then he said to the tree, "May no one ever eat fruit from you again." And his disciples heard him say it.

'In the morning, as they went along, they saw the fig tree withered from the roots. Peter remembered and said, "Rabbi, look! The tree you cursed has withered!" "Have faith in God." Jesus said. "I tell you the truth, if anyone says to this mountain, 'Go, throw yourself in the sea,' and does not doubt in his heart but believes that what he says will happen, it will be done for him. So I tell you, whatever you ask for in prayer, believe you have received it, and it will be yours. When you pray, if you hold anything against anyone, forgive them, so that your father in heaven may forgive you your sins."' – **Mark 11:12-26**

34. Jesus cursed a fig tree

As Jesus walked from Bethany to Jerusalem in Holy Week, he was hungry. He saw a fig tree and went to eat some of its fruit. When Jesus found none on the tree, he cursed it, vowing it would never bear fruit again. Mark 11:20 says that when the disciples saw the tree the next day, it was withered from the roots. The event reveals the power of Jesus' word. He cursed the tree and it died. It is how powerful his word is. He speaks and it happens. Also it reveals his divinity. He is God and the Creator of all things. When the Creator cursed his creation, the fig tree died. However, that is not how a tree usually dies. When a tree dies, death begins in the leaves then works through the branches into the trunk then down into the roots. It shows that the withering of this fig tree was supernatural and Matthew 21:19 confirms it by saying that the tree withered immediately. It is the power of Jesus Christ, the God of all creation and the power of his word.

This miracle is a parable

Cursing the fig tree seems harsh. However, it is another example of Jesus' miracle being a parable. The fig tree was the symbol of the nation Israel – the nation God had chosen out of the world to be His people – the people of God. Like a fig tree, it gave the appearance to the world it was fruitful – that it was a religious society that obeyed and served God. However, just as Jesus went to the tree and found no fruit, God came to Earth in human form and went to his people Israel, but he found no fruit. The people and their leaders were not obeying God but were serving themselves. At the Creation, God created the trees with seed bearing fruit to be food for mankind. But when the Creator (Jesus) came to his creation (the fig tree) and found it was not fulfilling its God-given purpose (to bear fruit), it was symbolic of God's people. He found they were not fulfilling the purpose for which He had chosen them. Worse still, when they rejected Jesus, their Creator, they became cursed like the fig tree. But those who believe he is God are like trees whose leaves are green and bear fruit in season (Psalm 1:1-3).

Have faith!

When the disciples asked Jesus how the fig tree had withered so quickly, he told them to have faith (Mark 11:22). He did not want them (and us) just speaking words of faith, he wanted them and us to believe in our hearts – to believe what God says in His word would happen. This is the grasping of God's promises that is the victory that has overcome the world, even our faith (1 John 5:4). He who believes that Jesus is the Christ overcomes the world. Faith comes by hearing and hearing by the words of Christ (Romans 10:17). Can there be anything easier? Faith enables us to lay hold of what is (sickness) and get it out of the way for God to bring in something that is not (healing).

God has given us this wonderful word. We have this word. *'We do not have to go up to highest heavens to bring God down or go down to the deepest depths to bring God up. His word is near us. It is in our mouths and in our hearts – that is the word we are proclaiming'* (Romans 10:6). We must believe that Jesus took our sins and bore them away in his body when he died on the cross. We must believe he was buried for us and that when he arose it was for us. Now Jesus sits at the right hand of God for us. If we can believe this in our hearts and confess with our mouths Jesus, the Son of God is Lord, then we are saved.

There is a rest of faith where we can put all of our trust in God and His word. It is the place where we believe that His promises never fail. Faith comes by hearing and hearing by the word of God (Romans 10:17). God's word can create in us an irresistible faith that is never daunted, never gives up and never fails. We must never fail to realise the abundance of God's inexhaustible supply. It pleases God when we ask for much and take much. The Feeding of the Five Thousand and the Feeding of the Four Thousand show that the more we take – the more we leave behind. When we ask God, we must believe that He will give us what we ask for (Mark 11:24). We just need to ask, believing that God will give it to us then receive it.

There are times in life when there seems to be a stone wall in front of us. Everything is black and there is nothing left – the doctors have said there is no cure – the debtors are about to take the family home – the love of our life is leaving – relationships are broken beyond repair – the shame of what we have done is unbearable. At these times in life, our confidence in God is the only thing we have left. Despite all that we see and are experiencing, we must be bold to believe that our heavenly Father will not fail and cannot fail.

We cannot depend on our feelings, but on His word. A divine revelation comes within us when we are born from above and it is real faith. To be born into His kingdom is to be born into a new faith. There is a big difference between our faith and Jesus' faith and his faith is in us. When Jesus cursed the fig tree, it withered from the roots. Just like this miracle was a parable for the religious leaders and the people of Israel, it is a parable for us as well. At times, Jesus will attack the roots of the sickness or disease or other problems in our lives. Only when the roots of our sickness, disease or problems have been destroyed will our healing or the resolution of our problem manifest itself in the physical.

Miracle 35

Jesus healed a man's ear

'While he was still speaking a crowd came up, and the man who was called Judas, one of the Twelve, was leading them. He approached Jesus to kiss him, but Jesus asked him, "Judas, are you betraying the Son of Man with a kiss?"

When Jesus' followers saw what was going to happen, they said, "Lord, should we strike with our swords?" And one of them struck the servant of the high priest, cutting off his right ear.

But Jesus answered, "No more of this!" And he touched the man's ear and healed him.

Then Jesus said to the chief priests, the officers of the temple guard, and the elders, who had come for him, "Am I leading a rebellion that you have come with swords and clubs? Every day I was with you in the temple courts, and you did not lay a hand on me. But this is your hour, when darkness reigns." **– Luke 22:47-53**

35. Jesus healed a man's ear

After Judas betrayed Jesus in Gethsemane, the soldiers stepped forward to arrest him. John 18:10 says Peter drew his sword and lashed out. He struck the ear of the servant of the high priest and severed it. His name was, 'Malchus,' which means, 'kingdom'. These happenings also reflected the spiritual state of the nation of Israel. When Jesus Christ the Son of God, the Saviour of the World was arrested, the ear of the kingdom of Israel was cut off. When the Hebrews rejected their Messiah – when they set in process the handing over of God's Son to the Gentiles to be killed, the subjects of the kingdom of Israel lost their hearing. They became deaf to the truths of the kingdom of God. They became deaf to the truths of Jesus Christ, God's Son, their redeemer and the Saviour of the World.

Matthew 26:50-54 and Mark 14:47 both record that one of Jesus' disciples cut off the ear of the high priest's servant with a sword, but only Luke records Jesus healed the man's severed ear. This account reveals his great compassion and love, even to those who hated him. It is easy to love those who love us. However, in this miracle Jesus demonstrated his great love and character. He practised what he preached; *'love your enemies'* (Matthew 5:44). He behaved the same towards his enemies as he did towards his friends by healing those who needed it. What a wonderful Saviour we have in Jesus.

Also, this healing is good news for the nation of Israel. The fact that Jesus healed Malchus' ear lets the people of Israel know that a time will come when God restores their hearing and the nation will hear the Good News of the Gospel of Jesus and will receive salvation. When the full number of the Gentiles has come into God's kingdom then Israel's hearing will be restored – Praise God!

Miracle 36

A miraculous catch of fish

'*Afterward Jesus appeared again to his disciples, by the Sea of Tiberius. It happened this way: Simon Peter, Thomas (called Didymus), Nathanael from Cana in Galilee, the sons of Zebedee, and two other disciples were together. "I'm going out to fish," Simon Peter told them, and they said, "We'll go with you." So they went out and got into the boat, but that night they caught nothing.*

Early in the morning, Jesus stood on the shore, but the disciples did not realise that it was Jesus.

He called out to them, "Friends, haven't you any fish?" "No," they answered. He said, "Throw your net on the right side of the boat and you will find some." When they did, they were unable to haul the net in because of the large number of fish.

Then the disciple whom Jesus loved said to Peter, "It is the Lord!" As soon as he heard him say, "It is the Lord," he wrapped his outer garment around him (for he had taken it off) and jumped into the water. The others followed in the boat, towing the net full of fish, for they were not far from shore, about a hundred yards. When they landed, they saw a fire of burning coals with fish on it, and some bread. Jesus said, "Bring some of the fish you have just caught." Simon climbed aboard and dragged the net ashore. It was full of large fish (one hundred and fifty-three), but even with so many the net was not torn. Jesus said to them, "Come and have breakfast." None of them dared ask him, "Who are you?" They knew it was the Lord.

Jesus came, took the bread and gave it to them, and did the same with the fish. This was now the third time Jesus had appeared to his disciples after he rose from the dead.

When they had finished eating, Jesus said to Simon Peter, "Simon, son of John, do you truly love me more than these?" He said, "Yes, Lord, you know that I love you." Jesus said, "Feed my lambs."

Again Jesus said, "Simon, son of John, do you truly love me?" He answered, "Yes, Lord, you know that I love you." Jesus said, "Take care of my sheep."

The third time he said to him, "Simon, son of John, do you love me?" Peter was hurt because he asked him the third time, "Do you love me?" He said, "Lord, you know all things; you know that I love you."

Jesus said, "Feed my sheep. I tell you the truth, when you were younger you dressed yourself and went where you wanted to go; but when you are old you will stretch out your hands, and someone else will dress you and lead you where you do not want to go. Jesus said this to indicate the kind of death by which Peter would glorify God. Then he said to him, "Follow me!"

Peter turned and saw the disciple whom Jesus loved following them. (This was the one who had leaned back against Jesus at the supper and had said, "Lord, who is going to betray you?") When Peter saw him, he asked, "Lord, what about him?"

Jesus answered, "If I want him to remain alive until I return, what is that to you? You must follow me!"

Because of this the rumour spread that this disciple would not die. But Jesus did not say that he would not die; he only said, "If I want him to remain alive until I return, what is that to you?" **– John 21:1-23**

36. A miraculous catch of fish

Peter was reinstated in his ministry by Jesus at the same place (the Sea of Galilee) and in the same circumstance (after a miraculous catch of fish) as when he was initially called to ministry when Jesus told him leave everything and follow him (Luke 5:1-11). When Jesus rose from the dead on the third day after his crucifixion, he told his disciples to go to Galilee, where they would see him (Matthew 28:10). So the disciples went to Galilee. Whilst they were waiting there to see Jesus, Peter and six others spent the night fishing on the lake, but caught nothing. That night they went out in Peter's timing, not Jesus' timing and they experienced an unsuccessful night of fishing. This reveals that when we go out in life without Jesus, when we act in our own timing and do not wait for God's timing, our 'nets' in life will be empty.

After a night of failure, Jesus, their Lord and Saviour came into the scene and the dynamics totally changed. He told them to drop their net on the right side of the boat for a catch of fish. Despite working all night and catching nothing, they obeyed Jesus' words. When they did, they caught such a large number of fish that they were unable to haul the net into the boat (John 21:6). Again Jesus showed his disciples (and us) his divinity and the inexhaustible, abundant supply of the kingdom of God. This is life in his kingdom. When we receive Jesus as Lord and Saviour and submit all that we are and all that we have to Jesus, our nets in life will be filled to bursting.

That day, on the Sea of Galilee, despite the abundance of Jesus' provision the disciples' net was not torn (John 21:11). And it is the same for us when Jesus pours the inexhaustible abundant supply of the kingdom of God into our lives – it will not destroy our bodies or our lives. He will expand our spirit, souls, bodies and lives to receive his abundance. As we rest in him and trust in him and his timing, this abundance will continue to be poured into our lives. This miracle shows we must wait on Jesus and trust in him and his timing then we will always be in the right place at the right time for the right thing.

Peter's growth

This second miraculous catch of fish on the Sea of Galilee marks the growth in Peter's story. At the first miraculous catch of fish he fell at Jesus' feet and begged him to go away from him as Peter recognised his own sinfulness and Jesus' holiness. It frightened him. At this last miraculous catch of fish, Peter still recognised his own sinfulness – he had recently abandoned Jesus when he was arrested then had denied him three times. But, when John told him that it was Jesus standing on the shore of the lake, Peter leapt out of the boat and hurried to him. His behaviour was so different from the first time Jesus provided him with a miraculous catch of fish. That time Peter pushed Jesus away. This time he ran to him. After three and half years of following Jesus and seeing him die on the cross of Calvary and rise to life again on the third day, Peter realised that not only was Jesus still holy, but also, he had only love for sinners (enough to die for them). That is why Peter hurried to Jesus. He knew he was loved and accepted, flaws and all.

Seeing in love

After Peter had spent the night fishing, the next day he was unable to recognise Jesus, his risen Lord standing on the shore. When Jesus provided Peter and the other disciples with a miracle catch of fish, it was John who was the first to recognise him. There is an interesting contrast here between Peter and John. On the night Jesus was betrayed, Peter trusted in his own love for the Lord to get him through what lay ahead. He boasted to Jesus that if all the others fell away, he would stand by him, even if it meant going to prison or even death. He believed his love and loyalty to Jesus was so strong, he would never fail Jesus, yet just hours later, he deserted him and denied him three times. John however trusted in Jesus' love for him, to such a level, he based his identity on it and called himself, 'the disciple whom Jesus loved' (John 13:24; John 19:26; John 20:2; John 21:7 and John 21:20). It was John who lived in the knowledge of Jesus' love, who was first to recognise his risen Lord standing by the Sea of Galilee that morning and not Peter who had trusted in his own love for Jesus.

Jesus turned bad memories to good memories

When Peter came ashore, there was risen Jesus standing by a fire of burning coals. The last time Peter had seen a fire of burning coals was when he denied Jesus three times in the courtyard of the high priest's palace on the night before he was crucified (Luke 22:54-62). It was just hours after Peter had vowed undying love and loyalty to Jesus. However, when Jesus looked at him with such love after the rooster crowed following his third denial of Jesus, it broke Peter.

It was a memory that haunted him until the day he saw Jesus standing by a fire of burning coals on the shore of the Sea of Galilee. Then he saw the one he had deserted and betrayed before he died on the cross was now alive for ever. What a joyous sight for Peter to behold. At this appearance, Jesus took what had been a terrible memory for Peter and turned it into a wonderful one. What selfless love Jesus showed him. And Jesus shows the same selfless love to us. He will take the worst thing that has happened in our lives and turn it into the best thing that has happened in our lives – if we let him.

Jesus provides for all of our needs

Not only was Jesus standing by a fire of burning coals, but also, he was cooking fish on them for their breakfast. Fish was what Peter and the six other disciples had spent the whole night looking for in order to feed themselves. Jesus was showing his disciples he has and would always have what they were looking for in life. Also it showed them he was able and would always be able to provide for their needs – even down to providing them breakfast. Jesus is the same today as he was that day by the lake. He always has what we are looking for in life and his inexhaustible, abundant supply will always meet our needs no matter how big or small they are. In God's kingdom we will find that healing is one of the many needs that Jesus, the king of the kingdom provides for his children. And these miracles are recorded in the Bible to encourage us to always come to Jesus, our Great Provider for all things, including the healing of our bodies, minds, souls and spirits.

153 fish

When Jesus told the disciples to throw their net on the right side of the boat they were unable to haul the net into the boat because of the large number of fish – 153. Numbers in the Bible always have a significance. The number, 153 is no exception. There is a message for us today in this number. If all the numbers contained in the sequence of numbers from one to seventeen (that is one + two + three, up to seventeen) are added together, then the total comes to one hundred and fifty-three:

1+2+3+4+5+6+7+8+9+10+11+12+13+14+15+16+17 = 153

Seventeen is the Hebrew number of **victory**. There is victory in Christ Jesus. This is the victory he won when he died on the cross of Calvary and rose on the third day. He rose victorious over death. He trampled death under his feet. Because Jesus defeated death, he defeated all sickness and disease as well as all the powers of evil and darkness. Because Jesus is victorious over death and all things, we can go to him when we need healing knowing that his victory on the cross of Calvary and over the grave guarantees our healing. It is all Jesus and what he has done for us on the cross – so the glory is all his. All we have to do is believe in Jesus Christ our crucified Lord and risen Saviour.

This is the last miracle recorded in the Gospels. The Gospels sign off in victory. It reveals to us that we will always have victory in Christ Jesus from beginning to end. All things in heaven and on Earth are under Jesus' authority. So we will not just have victory in one or two things. We will have victory in all things. What a wonderful Saviour we have in Jesus Christ our Lord – all praise and glory to God!

Jesus healed the crowds

For over three years Jesus preached the good news of God's kingdom, healed the sick and drove out demons. John 21:25 says if all his miracles were recorded, the world would not have enough room for all the books. The Gospels record just thirty-six of them. But there were many times when he healed the people en-masse:

A. At the Passover Feast after his baptism

'While he was in Jerusalem at the Passover, many people saw the miracles he was doing and believed in his name.' – **John 2:23**

'Nicodemus came to Jesus at night saying, "Rabbi, we know you are a teacher who has come from God. For no one could perform the miracles you are doing if God were not with him."' – **John 3:2**

B. As he began his Galilean ministry

'Jesus went throughout Galilee, teaching in their synagogues; preaching the good news of the kingdom, and healing every disease and sickness among the people.' – **Matthew 4:23**

C. Before the Sermon on the Mount

'News about him spread all over Syria and people brought to him all who were ill with various diseases, those suffering severe pain, the demon-possessed, those having seizures, and the paralysed, and he healed them.' – **Matthew 4:24**

'When they heard all he was doing, many people came to him from Judea, Jerusalem, Idumea, and the regions across the Jordan and around Tyre and Sidon. Because of the crowd, he told his disciples to have a small boat ready for him, to keep the people from crowding him. For he had healed many, so that those with diseases were pushing forward to touch him. Whenever the evil spirits saw him, they fell down before him and cried out, "You are the Son of God." But he gave them strict orders not to tell who he was' – **Mark 3:8-12**

'*A large crowd of disciples was there and a great number of people from Judea, Jerusalem, and from the coast of Tyre and Sidon who had come to hear him and be healed of their diseases. Those troubled by evil spirits were cured and the people all tried to touch him, as power was coming from him and healing them all.*' – **Luke 6:17-19**

D. When John's disciples came to Jesus

'*Jesus replied, "Go back and report to John what you hear and see: 'The blind receive sight, the lame walk, those who have leprosy are cured, the deaf hear, the dead are raised, and the good news is preached to the poor. Blessed is the man who does not fall away on account of me."*' – **Matthew 11:4-5**

'*At that very time Jesus cured many who had diseases, sicknesses and evil spirits and gave sight to many who were blind. So he replied to the messengers, "Go back and report to John what you have seen and heard: The blind receive sight, the lame walk, those who have leprosy are cured, the deaf hear, the dead are raised, and the good news is preached to the poor. Blessed is the man who does not fall away on account of me."*' – **Luke 7:21-23**

E. Before Jesus taught the crowds in parables

'*After this, Jesus went about from one town and village to another, proclaiming the good news of the kingdom of God. The Twelve were with him and also some women who had been cured of evil spirits and diseases. Mary (called Magdalene) from whom seven demons had come out; Joanna, the wife of Cuza, the manager of Herod's household; Susanna and many others.*' – **Luke 8:1-3**

F. Before Jesus sent out the twelve apostles

'*Jesus went through all the towns and villages teaching in their synagogues, preaching the good news of the kingdom, healing every disease and sickness.*' – **Matthew 9:35**

G. Before Jesus fed the Five Thousand

'When Jesus landed and saw a large crowd he had compassion on them and healed their sick.' – **Matthew 14:14**

'Then he took them with him and they withdrew by themselves to a town called Bethsaida, but the crowds learned about it and followed him. He welcomed them and spoke to them about the kingdom of God, and he healed those who needed healing.' – **Luke 9:10-11**

H. After Jesus walked on water

'And when the men of that place recognised Jesus, they sent word to all the surrounding country. People brought all their sick to him and begged him to let the sick just touch the edge of his cloak, and all who touched him were healed.' – **Matthew 14:35-36**

'They ran throughout that whole region and carried the sick on mats to wherever they heard he was. And wherever he went – into villages, towns or countryside – they placed the sick in the marketplaces. They begged him to let them touch even the edge of his cloak, and all who touched him were healed.' – **Mark 6:55-56**

I. Before Jesus fed the Four Thousand

'Great crowds came to him bringing the lame, the blind, the crippled, the mute and many others and laid them at his feet; and he healed them. The people were amazed when they saw the mute speaking; the crippled made well; the lame walking and the blind seeing. And they praised the God of Israel.' – **Matthew 15:30-31**

J. In Judea across the Jordan

'When Jesus had finished saying these things, he left Galilee and went into the region of Judea to the other side of the Jordan. Large crowds followed him and he healed them there.' – **Matthew 19:1-2**

All Jesus' miracles and healings to individuals and the crowds are:

All of Jesus' healings and miracles
Early ministry
1 Jesus turned water into wine at Cana
A **Jesus did miracles at the Passover Feast in Jerusalem**
2 Jesus healed a royal official's son in Cana
Jesus' first year of ministry
3 Miraculous catch of fish on the Sea of Galilee
4 Sabbath healing of a demoniac in Capernaum
5 Sabbath healing of Peter's Mother-in-law in Capernaum
6 Jesus healed all the sick and demonised in Capernaum
7 Jesus healed a leper in Galilee
B **Jesus healed the crowds who came to him in Galilee**
8 Jesus healed a paralytic at Peter's home in Capernaum
Jesus' second year of ministry
9 Sabbath healing of a man's hand in Capernaum
C **Crowds healed before the Sermon on the Mount**
10 Jesus healed a centurion's servant in Capernaum
11 Jesus raised a widow's only son from the dead at Nain
D **Crowds healed in front of John's disciples**
12 Jesus healed a blind, mute demoniac in Capernaum
E **Crowds healed before Jesus taught in parables**
13 Jesus calmed a storm on the Sea of Galilee
14 Jesus healed two demoniacs in the Gadarenes
15 Jesus healed a bleeding woman in Capernaum
16 Jesus raised Jairus' daughter in Capernaum
17 Jesus healed two blind men in Capernaum
18 Jesus healed a mute demoniac in Capernaum
19 Sabbath healing of a paralytic at a feast in Jerusalem
F **Jesus healed in Israel then sent out the Twelve**
G **Crowds healed before Jesus fed the Five Thousand**
20 Jesus fed the Five Thousand by the Sea of Galilee
21 Jesus walked on the Sea of Galilee
H **Jesus healed the crowds in Galilee**

Jesus' final year of ministry
22 Jesus healed a woman's demonised daughter in Tyre
23 Jesus healed a deaf mute in the Decapolis
I **Crowds healed before Jesus fed the Four Thousand**
24 Jesus fed the Four Thousand by the Sea of Galilee
25 Jesus healed a blind man at Bethsaida
26 Sabbath healing of a blind man in Jerusalem
27 Jesus raised Lazarus from the dead at Bethany
28 Jesus healed a father's demonised son
29 The coin in the fish's mouth in the Sea of Galilee
J **Jesus healed the crowds in Judea across the Jordan**

Jesus' final journey to Jerusalem
30 Jesus healed ten lepers on the Galilee-Samaria border
31 Sabbath healing of a crippled woman in a synagogue
32 Sabbath healing of a man with dropsy in a leader's home
33 Jesus healed two blind men at Jericho

Jesus' final Passover in Jerusalem
34 Jesus cursed a fig tree at Bethany in Judea
35 Jesus healed a man's severed ear in Gethsemane

After the Resurrection
36 Miraculous catch of fish on the Sea of Galilee

The abundance of Jesus' healing

The Gospels reveal Jesus healed in abundance, be it individuals or crowds. He provided an abundance of vintage wine at the wedding in Cana. Many Jews saw all the miracles he did at the Passover. He provided a net-breaking, boat-sinking haul of fish for Peter. He healed all the sick and demonised in Capernaum, making it a sick-free town. He made Galilee a sick-free region by healing every disease and sickness in all of its towns and villages. People came from everywhere to hear Jesus' words and power came out of him and healed them all. John the Baptist's disciples saw Jesus heal many diseased, sick, blind and demonised people. Then Jesus travelled through all of Israel healing every disease and sickness.

Jesus healed all the sick before he fed the Five Thousand and the Four Thousand. Everyone was filled and there was an abundance of leftovers. Between the two miracle feedings, wherever he went, all the sick who touched him were healed. Large crowds followed Jesus over the Jordan and he healed them all. He continued to heal people on his final journey to Jerusalem. Days after arriving in the capital, Jesus the Son of God gave his all when he died for our sins. And by his stripes we are healed of all diseases and sicknesses.

Oh, the abundance of Jesus and the kingdom of God. He healed all who came to him of every disease and sickness. His abundant power delivered demoniacs, whether they were possessed by one or a thousand evil spirits. Three times his abundant compassion raised the dead to life. He healed and delivered in all the towns and villages of Galilee and Israel. There was no one who came to him that he did not heal and there was no disease he was unable to heal – even death. Healing people – be it crowds or individuals was part of his daily life here on Earth. Jesus is the same today as he was yesterday and will be forever. Healing is who he is. It was then and it is now. If Jesus was willing and able to heal people of their diseases and sicknesses in their day then we must see that he is just as willing and able to heal us of all our diseases and sicknesses today when we come to him to be healed.

Jesus was not only willing to heal a leper; he was willing to touch him. He was always full of compassion to those who came to him. He had compassion on the crowds whom he saw as lost sheep without a shepherd. He had compassion on individuals, like the bleeding woman, the man with the shrivelled hand, the woman who had been crippled for eighteen years and the man who had been paralysed for thirty-eight years. All these people were on the fringes of society, excluded from religious life until the source of their faith came and healed them. Jesus embraced the man with dropsy to heal him and his arms are open wide today to embrace all who seek healing. Come to Jesus and be healed!

The ways Jesus healed

The power and authority of his words

The authority and power of Jesus' word cast out demons, diseases and fevers throughout his ministry. By his word: the blind saw; the deaf heard; mutes spoke; the lame walked; lepers were cleansed; and paralytics and the dead were raised. His all powerful word transcends time and distance. It changes that which is not, into that which is (water into wine, death into life, sickness into health, blindness into sight, deafness into hearing and lack into abundance). Jesus' word had the power to heal all diseases and sicknesses then and it has the same power to heal all our diseases and sicknesses today.

Obedience to Jesus' words

Obedience to Jesus' word produced miracles. Water became wine as slaves obeyed him and filled the jars with water and served it. When Jesus told the official to go home, he obeyed and found his son well. Peter obeyed Jesus' words and experienced two miraculous catches of fish and walked on water. One word from Jesus and demons fled, be it one or a thousand. In obedience to Jesus' word, leprosy, paralysis, sickness, disease, blindness and even death departed. What a Saviour we have in Jesus Christ our Lord! That power is available to everyone today when we are obedient to his sovereign word.

The created obeyed its Creator

Whenever Jesus cast out demons, the created obeyed its Creator. Creation obeyed its Creator when he calmed the storm and when the fig tree withered. At his word, shoals of fish twice swam into Peter's nets on the lake and on one occasion every fish swam out of the way to let the fish with a coin in its mouth bite on Peter's hook. At his word, water became wine at a wedding. Twice, at his word, his disciples fed thousands of people until they were full with just a few loaves and a few fish. At Jesus' word, the supernatural triumphed over the natural as the impossible occurred. And it still occurs today.

The power of Jesus' touch

Jesus healed the sick and diseased with a touch or by laying his hands on them. When he touched Peter's mother-in-law's hand the fever left her and she got up from her bed. He healed all the sick in Capernaum by laying hands on them. Jesus healed a blind man by spitting in his eyes and touching them. He healed a man with dropsy by laying hold of him. He healed Caiaphas' servant's ear with a touch.

Jesus healed others with a touch and a word. He raised Jairus' daughter by taking her by the hand and telling her to get up. He healed a deaf mute by putting his fingers in his ears, touching his tongue and saying, "be opened!" Jesus healed a blind man by putting mud in his eyes and telling him to go and wash in the Pool of Siloam. Jesus healed a crippled woman by laying hands on her and telling her she was free from her infirmity. His touch was all powerful when he ministered here on Earth and his touch is just as powerful today. Reach out and let the Lord Jesus Christ touch you and heal you.

Healed by faith

Jesus commended all who came to him in faith to be healed. When he saw the faith of the four men carrying their paralysed friend on a stretcher, he healed the man. After seeing a centurion's 'great faith,' Jesus healed his paralysed servant. He praised a woman who had bled for twelve years when she touched the edge of his cloak in faith to be healed. He responded to two blind men's faith in Capernaum by restoring their sight. When a mother showed "great faith", Jesus healed her demon-possessed daughter. He commended the faith of the man he had healed of leprosy who returned to thank him for his healing. Then he healed two blind men at Jericho according to their faith. Like all these people, when we come to Jesus in faith he will give us all that we ask for. As Peter fixed his eyes on Jesus, the supernatural occurred and he walked on water. As we fix our eyes on Jesus Christ, the Son of God, who is God and not on ourselves or on our symptoms, then the supernatural will occur in our lives as well.

Power to heal

The power to replace the visible (sickness) with the invisible (health) was not only in Jesus' words and his touch. There were times when the power to heal was present with him, as in the case of the paralytic he healed in Capernaum. Power came out of Jesus to heal the crowds before the Sermon on the Mount and to heal the woman who had bled for twelve years in Capernaum. Jesus was and is full of healing power. It exuded from him then and it exudes from him now. He was so full of healing power that it saturated his clothing. All a person who needing healing had to do was touch it. Today, Jesus is just as full of healing power as he was then and all we need to do is reach out and touch even the edge of his cloak and we too will be healed. Jesus' love, compassion, willingness and power to heal are far greater than any disease or sickness, no matter how long it has been there – be it twelve years (like the bleeding woman) or eighteen years (like the crippled woman) or thirty-eight years (like the paralytic in Jerusalem).

Thanking God produced miracles

Miracles occurred after Jesus thanked his heavenly Father. When he fed the Five Thousand and the Four Thousand, he took the loaves of bread and the fish and thanked God before giving it to his disciples to distribute to the people. As a result, everyone was fed to the full and there were baskets of leftovers. Jesus thanked God for hearing him before he raised Lazarus. We too must thank God when we ask Him for healing and not just after we have received it.

Love and compassion to heal

At the heart of Jesus' healing ministry was and is his great love and his great compassion. Time and again he showed his and his heavenly Father's love to heal the sick. In great compassion he reached out to touch a leper to heal him. His compassion was greater than death, which had to give back the widow's only son, Jairus' twelve year-old daughter and Mary and Martha's brother, Lazarus. And out of his great love and great compassion, Jesus healed and fed the crowds.

Jesus raises us up and restores us

During his ministry Jesus always raised people up. He took Peter's mother-in-law by the hand and raised her up. He raised up three paralytics, two in Capernaum and one in Jerusalem. He raised up three dead people: a widow's son, Jairus' daughter and Lazarus. He took the widow's son and gave him back to his mother. He took Jairus' daughter by the hand and gave her back to her parents. This is Jesus and life in God's kingdom where people are restored to health and families are restored as well. He loved to restore children to their parents. He did it when he healed the official's son, the demonised daughter of a Syro-Phoenician woman and the demonised son of an anguished father. This is Jesus and his kingdom. In it, sickness, disease, evil and death are defeated and lives and families are restored and made whole.

Knowing our standing and our status

As Jesus healed people, he restored their standing and status as well. He told a paralytic, "*Son, your sins are forgiven.*" By calling him, 'Son,' he restored his standing as he declared the man was a son of Abraham and a child of God – such a loving and affirmative declaration. After restoring his standing, Jesus restored his status by saying his sins were forgiven. The paralytic needed to know that his sins were forgiven in order to receive his healing. Once his status and standing had been restored, he stood physically. Out of his great love and compassion, Jesus, the Son of God healed this man completely – at all levels.

Jesus did the same when he healed a crippled woman. After healing her physically, he restored her standing by calling her, 'daughter of Abraham.' He was stating she was as much a Jew and a child of God as everyone else in the synagogue that day. Jesus did the same thing when he called a bleeding woman, 'daughter.' Jesus did not want these suffering people identifying themselves by their illness. He wanted them to know he was not condemning them for their sin. He took their eyes off their illness and sinfulness and fixed them on him.

Jesus is the same yesterday, today and forever. The same love, compassion, authority and power that healed and delivered all who came to him whilst he was here on Earth is available to all who come to him today. He longs to raise us up from our sickbeds and deliver us from all that oppresses us and restore our standing and status. He yearns to restore all that has been lost in every area of our lives. He wants to raise us up into the fullness of life that he came to bring and is freely available to everyone in his kingdom. He wants us to know that he is not condemning us for our sins and wants us to live in the fullness of our standing in him. The Gospels help us believe Jesus does not condemn us when they record no occasion during his ministry when he condemned anyone for their sins when they came to him to be healed.

All we need to do to receive Jesus' healing and all his goodness in our lives is acknowledge we need a saviour – and Jesus is the only Saviour: *'Salvation is found in no one else, for there is no other name under heaven given to men by which we must be saved'* (Acts 4:12). Then we are restored to our full standing and status in him. When we know who we are in Christ, we receive all God has given us in him. Before we can know who we are, we need to know whose we are. When we believe in Jesus, we become children of God (John 1:12-13) and belong to God. All the words He spoke about His children apply to us. Because Jesus died on the cross for us, God sees us in Christ as pure, forgiven, washed, holy, righteous and free from all the curses of our fallen state, especially sickness, disease and oppression.

On the cross of Calvary, Jesus became our sin and we became his righteousness. We did not deserve to become his righteousness just as much as he did not deserve to become our sin. But it is the benefit of the covenant God made with Jesus – the Lamb of God gave his life for our sins. This New Covenant was between God and Jesus (not God and the Devil) to break the powers of darkness in people's lives. Because of God's great love in sending His Son Jesus to die for us, we become the beneficiaries of this New Covenant.

When Jesus is our Lord and Saviour, we become beneficiaries of this covenant. Like a beneficiary of a will, the only qualification to benefit from it, is to be born into the dead person's family. When we are born again, we are born into our heavenly Father's family and inherit all the benefits from Jesus' death. We did not participate in the agreeing and fulfilling of this covenant, so there is nothing we can do or say to change its terms and conditions. In this New Covenant between God and Jesus, we, the beneficiaries are loved by God. There is nothing we can do or say or not do or not say to make God love us any more or any less. We are righteous, holy, pure and spotless in God's sight because of Jesus' finished work on the cross of Calvary.

We are right with God (Romans 8:1), we have peace with God and we have the peace of God – because of Jesus' finished work on the cross. If we believe we have to do something to be saved and have peace with God, our salvation depends on us. If it depends on us, we do not need a saviour. There is nothing we can do to be saved. It is the gift of God and there is nothing we can do to lose it. The life Jesus gives is eternal. If we are born again we live forever. His death and resurrection were enough to redeem us completely from sin and free us from every disease and sickness and from all the powers of evil.

Our status and our standing are in Jesus

When we receive Jesus as our Lord and Saviour, we enter God's kingdom and become His children and receive all He has for us – including healing. He restores our status and standing to receive the fullness of life Jesus came to give. Look to Jesus our Saviour. Trust him. Rely on him and his love. He loves to save us, heal us and set us free from all that binds, mars and hinders us. He is more willing to help than we are to ask. The price is paid for all our sicknesses and diseases. Illness is not our status or standing in life. Our illness is not who we are. It is not our identity. We must see our true status and standing in Christ and take it. Then, like Jesus, we will give thanks for the miracle we are looking for in our lives before we receive it and believe we have received it when we ask for it.

We must fix our eyes on Jesus, not on our symptoms. We must trust in him and his words and not trust in ourselves. We may think we are not righteous enough, good enough or holy enough to receive anything from him, but we must not and cannot trust in ourselves. We must trust in Jesus' righteousness, goodness and holiness. It is he who makes us right with God by his shed blood. It is nothing we do. It is all God. His grace and power are limitless. To believers, all things are possible.

The Spirit of the Sovereign Lord is upon Jesus, because God anointed him to preach the good news to the poor; to bind up the broken-hearted; to deliver captives, give sight to the blind and to set the bound free (Luke 4:18-19). He heals the broken-hearted and lets captives go free today and saves the worst of people. The good news is that through Jesus, we have peace with God. It brings liberty. It brings our souls out of bondage and brings perfect health to our bodies. The Gospel brings complete salvation. We must let Jesus' blood cleanse us from all sin and have faith in Jesus and his name and his sacrifice on the cross. We must have faith that on the cross Jesus took all our weaknesses upon himself and bore our sicknesses and diseases away and by his stripes we are healed. He has everything for everybody: forgiveness of sins; healing of diseases and fullness of life. All of this comes from Jesus. Seek him now! Call on his name now!

All things are possible through the name of Jesus. God has highly exalted him and given him the name that is above every name. There is no other name under heaven given to men whereby we must be saved. There is power to overcome everything through Jesus' name. There is power in Jesus and his wondrous name to transform anyone and to heal anyone and to meet every condition of human need. If we will only see that Jesus is the Lamb of God who takes away the sins of the world. If only we will see Jesus as the beloved Son of God who had laid upon him the iniquity of us all. If only we will see he paid the whole price for our redemption that we might be free. Then we can enter into our purchased inheritance of salvation, healing, fullness of life and power and access to God our heavenly Father.

Healing for the believer

In the Bible, God gives clear instructions for those who belong to the Church of Jesus who need healing:

"'Is any one of you sick? He should call the elders of the church; and let them pray over him and anoint him with oil in the name of the Lord. And the prayer offered in faith will make the sick person well; and the Lord will raise him up. If he has sinned sin then he will be forgiven. Therefore confess you sins to each other and pray for each other so that you may be healed.'" – **James 5:14-16**

These verses tell us what the sick in the Church need to do to receive healing. The role of the sick person is to call the elders of their church. The role of the elders is to anoint the sick person with oil and pray over them, 'the Prayer of Faith'. So, if the sick person does their part – call the elders; and if the elders of the church do their part – anoint the sick person and pray in faith, the whole situation then rests with God, who will then do His part – raise them up. If the sick person has sinned, their sins are forgiven. When we have been anointed and prayed for, we can rest assured God will do His part. It is the word of God. It cannot be otherwise. God said it and He will do it. He has lain down the terms and conditions. And as God has said it, He will keep His end of it.

In God's kingdom there is an abundance of love and compassion to heal and to provide. There is an abundance of power to heal. There is an abundant willingness to heal. Healing is not just something that Jesus does, it is who he is. It is part of his character and nature. He heals because he is healing. Jesus is the Healer. In the same way Jesus is compassion and he is love. Love and compassion are his character and nature. It is who he is. We can fully trust the abundance of his compassion, love and healing will never fail. The more we take, the more we leave behind. There is no lack with Jesus. His supply of healing always, abundantly exceeds our demand for healing.

Listening and looking at Jesus

We can only receive from God by faith. We are saved by faith and are healed by faith. As Jesus is the author and finisher of faith, we receive faith by spending time with him and his word. *'Faith comes by hearing and hearing by the word of Christ.'* (Romans 10:17). 'Hearing' is repeated twice and is in the present continuous tense. It is not by having heard once; it is by continual hearing of the good news of the Gospel that we have peace with God due to Jesus' finished work on the cross of Calvary. God sees us as perfect, because He sees Jesus' perfect work in removing our sin. As we hear the word about God's goodness, love, compassion and power, faith comes.

Isaiah 55:3 says if we continually listen to His word, God will satisfy our souls with eternal life and fill them with the richest of fare. By listening to His word, He fills us, satisfying our souls with abundant life. Nothing else will do it. Exodus 15:26 says if we listen to His words continually and obey God, He will heal us. When Jesus became our sin on the cross, we became his righteousness. In that righteousness, all the righteous requirements of the Law were met in him. Because Jesus kept all of the Law, it is credited to our account, not because of what we have done, but because of what he did. As Jesus has kept the Law we receive all the benefits – including healing.

God's requirement for healing then was to keep on listening to His word and it still is today. When Jesus' ministry began, word about him spread and crowds came to him to listen and be healed (Luke 6:17-19). They received their healing after listening to him. And it is the same today. People who want healing have to hear. Faith is the response to God's goodness. If we need healing we must ensure we listen to all that God says on healing – be it through sermons in Church or reading the Bible. After we have heard or read God's word, we must meditate on it and quote the words to ourselves. We must not let His word depart from our mouths and we will have success (Joshua 1:8). The Holy Spirit will breathe on the word and make it Spirit and life and health to us.

Receive eternal life now

The greatest gift we can receive from God in Christ Jesus is not our healing, but eternal life. Jesus' death on the cross of Calvary makes this possible. If we will repent of our sins and turn from our sins and believe in him, then eternal life, healing, health and all the other things that his death achieved are ours. If you would like to receive all that Jesus has done for you as Lord and Saviour, pray this prayer:

Lord Jesus Christ, the Son of God, thank you for loving me and dying for me on the cross. Your precious blood washes me clean of every sin, past present and future. You are my Lord and Saviour, now and always. I believe when you died on the cross and were buried you bore away my sins, diseases, sicknesses and death. I believe you rose again and are alive today, reigning over all things at the right hand of God in heaven. You rose without my sins, diseases and sicknesses. Because of your finished work, I am now a beloved child of God and heaven is my home. All the promises of God are now mine in you Lord Jesus, including my deliverance and my healing. Thank you Lord for giving me eternal life and for filling me with the Holy Spirit and for filling me with your peace and joy. Amen

If you prayed this prayer or have been healed by reading this book, please tell someone at your local church and contact me at: thejesusdiary1@gmail.com

God bless you!

Other titles by John Maxwell

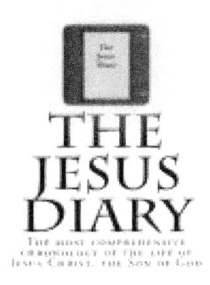

THE JESUS DIARY

THE CHRONOLOGY OF JESUS' LIFE – PART 1

'The Jesus Diary' is the most comprehensive chronology of events in the life of Jesus the Son of God ever written.

Jesus visited Earth at a point in time. The Gospels give four accounts of the one story of his birth, life, death and resurrection. *'The Jesus Diary'* is Part 1 of 'The Chronology of Jesus' Life' series. It puts events of his life in the order they occurred in history. The result is the most detailed chronology of his life ever written. It helps solidify the faith of believers and satisfies the curiosity of those who seek to know when God walked in human form on planet Earth. It is a great aid to pastors, preachers, and Bible students, as it reveals:

- The year Jesus was born and how long he spent in Egypt
- When Jesus was baptised and his ministry began
- When John the Baptist was killed and Jesus fed the 5,000
- The hour, the day and the year that Jesus died
- The dates Jesus rose again and ascended into heaven

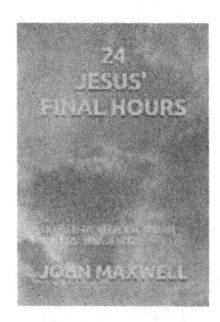

24 – JESUS' FINAL HOURS

THE CHRONOLOGY OF JESUS' LIFE – PART 2

For the first time, the final twenty-four hours of Jesus' life have been set into twenty-four, hour-by-hour sections

Twenty-four hours is one turn of the Earth on its axis. Most days blend into each other, but one day changed the world forever – The day Jesus the Son of God died. All events in history prior to it led to that point and all events since then have led from that point. *24 – Jesus' Final Hours* is Part 2 of 'The Chronology of Jesus' Life' series. It will change the way people see his death and the way they see the God who became man. The revelation of what he suffered to free me and all people from sin has inspired me to look at his death in even greater detail. Join me on this journey through Jesus' final hours and you will discover more of the sacrificial love and selfless, giving character of Jesus Christ the Son of God, who is God. Also, this book reveals:

- When the Last Supper in the Upper Room took place
- How long Jesus prayed for in the garden of Gethsemane
- The times of Jesus' trials and Peter's denials
- At what hour Jesus was crucified, died and was buried

40 DAYS OF RESURRECTION APPEARANCES
THE CHRONOLOGY OF JESUS' LIFE – PART 3

For the first time, the forty days of resurrection appearances are broken down into forty, day-by-day sections, which reveal:

- The number and order of Jesus' resurrection appearances
- How many people risen Jesus appeared to
- The significance of the locations where Jesus appeared
- The dates Jesus rose to life and ascended to heaven

'*40 Days of Resurrection Appearances*' is Part 3 of 'The Chronology of Jesus' Life' series. It takes an in-depth, day-by-day look at how his appearances break down into a forty-day period. It reveals when he appeared to his disciples and when he did not. There is as much to learn about Jesus and his disciples from the times when he did not appear to them as there is when he did appear to them. Join me on this day-by-day journey of forty days to find what Jesus' disciples learned from his appearances and absences and how that can be applied to our own lives today. It will change the way we view Jesus Christ and his resurrection and the way we view ourselves – forever!

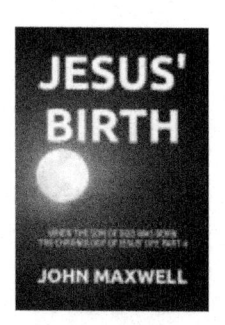

JESUS' BIRTH
THE CHRONOLOGY OF JESUS' LIFE – PART 4

A forensic examination of the information found in the Gospels regarding Jesus' birth to establish when God's Son was born.

'Jesus' Birth' is Part 4 of 'The Chronology of Jesus' Life' series. It not only establishes when Jesus was born, but it sets the existence of God on Earth in history using both Roman and Jewish historical records. Also, this book examines the 'missing years' between his birth and his baptism and what that means to us today. It reveals:

- The year Jesus was born and how long he was in Egypt
- The age difference between Jesus and John the Baptist
- When Jesus visited the temple in Jerusalem as a child
- What happened between Jesus' birth and his baptism

There is historical information in the Gospels for time of Jesus' birth until the time he was baptised. The writer has used the information and combined it with great numeracy skills to establish the year God's Son was born in human form on Earth. Enjoy this revealing read as it transforms your view of Jesus' birth, his existence and his deity.

NEW RELEASES by JOHN MAXWELL

HISTORICAL JESUS

'Historical Jesus' is the most comprehensive chronology of events in the ministry of Jesus, God's Son ever written.

Jesus, God's Son visited this Earth at a point in history. The Gospels give four accounts of the one story of Jesus' ministry. *'Historical Jesus'* sets all of the events of Jesus' ministry in the order they occurred and places each one on a specific date in history. From this most detailed chronology of events, the writer explores all the aspects of his ministry from a chronological perspective, which give great insights into Jesus' miracles, teachings, prayers, healings and the prophecies made about him. Also, it examines the main characters in Jesus' time of ministry and his relationships with those people.

Great tool for pastors, preachers and students

'Historical Jesus' helps pastors and preachers eliminate chronological inaccuracies from their sermons, which will increase the impact of their message. The book is a great study aid for Bible students as it reveals:

- The year Jesus was born and how long he spent in Egypt
- When Jesus was baptised and his Galilean ministry began
- When John the Baptist was killed and Jesus fed the 5,000
- The hour-by-hour breakdown of Jesus' final hours
- The exact times that Peter denied Jesus
- The dates Jesus died, rose again and ascended into heaven

An ideal gift for Church leaders

'Historical Jesus' is the ideal gift for pastors, leaders, preachers and lovers of the Bible as it contains a wealth of material useful for sermons and teaching. It will be a real blessing to all who receive it.

40 DAYS – JESUS' TEMPLATE FOR HIS CHURCH
HOW HE WANTS HIS CHURCH TO OPERATE

After Jesus rose from the dead, he appeared to his disciples over a period of forty days. At each appearance, he revealed different aspects of how his Church would operate.

'*40 Days of Resurrection Appearances*' looks at Jesus' appearances after he rose from the dead and reflects on the events of his time of ministry through his disciples' eyes after they witnessed him die and rise again. It reveals that at each appearances, he highlighted to them the elements to be included in Church services: worship, prayer, Holy Communion, miracles, prophecies, testimonies and sermons that revealed him in the Scriptures. It shows Jesus intended his Church to be a place where all are welcome to come to seek him and have their doubts listened to, and have those doubts turned to faith by patient, loving and caring leaders. It shows he intended his Church to be based on his words and all that is written about him in the Scriptures.

In the template of his Church, given to his disciples, Jesus intended it to be a place of love, joy, peace, healing, restoration, giving, praise, worship and prayer. A place where miracles, signs, and prophecies happened each time his people met. The meetings were to be so full of life and joy and revelation that all those present could not wait to share with others what they had experienced and learned about Jesus.

In the world today, some churches are not operating as Jesus intended. They need to return to Jesus' mandate for his Church. This book shows how he intended it to operate. When churches operate in the way he intended, they will be filled with people full of the joy of the Lord and the fullness of life Jesus came to bring them. Also the Church will have the full impact on the world that Jesus intended.

MY STORY, HIS GLORY

'My story, His Glory' is the testimony of the conversion of John Maxwell. In August 1994, John, who was not a Christian, went to church. He sat in a pew, disliking every minute of the experience and vowing never to go again when suddenly he felt a current of fire flow up and down his body. All his angst left him and a wonderful peace filled him. At the end of the service the first thing he said was, "I can't wait for next week." He entered the church vowing to never go again and left it eagerly looking ahead to the next service. That eagerness has never left him.

However, that was just the start of a set of extraordinary events that saw John prophesy a week later. Then he had dreams where he was taken up to heaven where he heard God both speak and laugh. After that, he had wonderful, supernatural encounters that could only have been orchestrated by God. He received wonderful words of knowledge to help others receive breakthroughs in their lives. The baptism of fire John received that day in St. Andrew's Church in Hong Kong during the movement of the Holy Spirit in the time of the Toronto Blessing is real and available to anyone who seeks it today.

If you hunger for that fire, join John as he looks at the supernatural events that took place around his conversion. It is journey that will encourage and inspire you to receive the Baptism of the Holy Spirit.

The ideal gift for those seeking salvation

'My Story, His Glory' is a great gift for anyone who is searching for God and eternal life or for a loved one with whom you want to share the good news about Jesus. It is the perfect reading companion for anyone doing the Alpha Course or any other basic Christianity course.

Available in hardback and paperback at Amazon.com and Amazon.co.uk

Printed in Great Britain
by Amazon